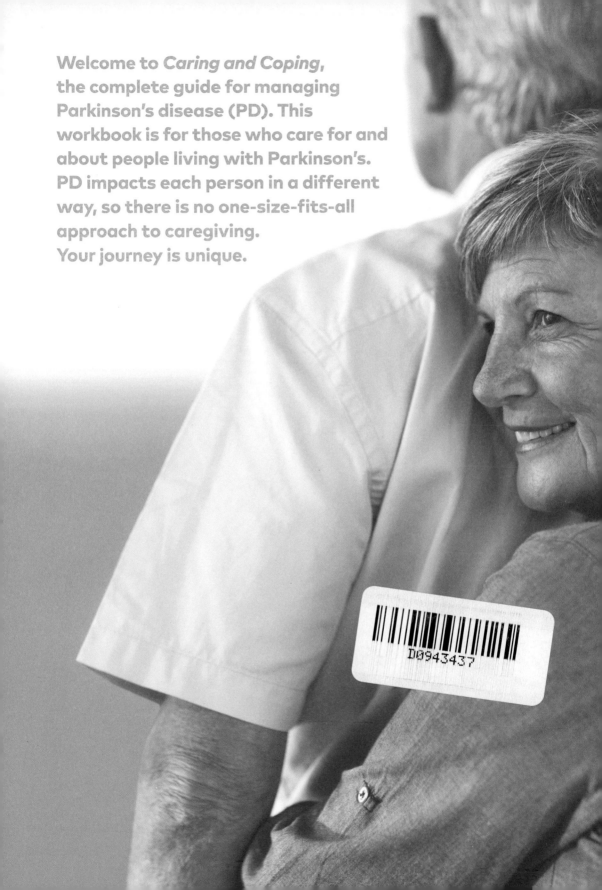

Welcome to *Caring and Coping*, the complete guide for managing Parkinson's disease (PD). This workbook is for those who care for and about people living with Parkinson's. PD impacts each person in a different way, so there is no one-size-fits-all approach to caregiving. Your journey is unique.

Introduction

Whether the Parkinson's diagnosis is new to your loved one or you have been living with Parkinson's for a long time, you have the right and responsibility to make the care partnership as productive as possible, with the least amount of stress and conflict. Preparation is key in all respects: emotional, financial and physical. We hope that the tips and tools in this workbook will help prepare you for every step of the journey.

WHAT IS CAREGIVING?

A precise definition remains elusive, despite growing numbers of people serving in the role of family caregiver. It is estimated that there are almost 45 million family caregivers in the United States, and more than three quarters of them care for someone over 50 years old.

A 2014 report from the National Alliance for Caregiving suggests the following definition: "Caregiving is everything we do to assist a friend or relative due to that person's illness or disability, and that we do for our own health." This book is focused on that dual role: you provide care for someone else – the "caring" part of *Caring and Coping*. Just as importantly, you also must take care of yourself – the "coping" portion of this book's title.

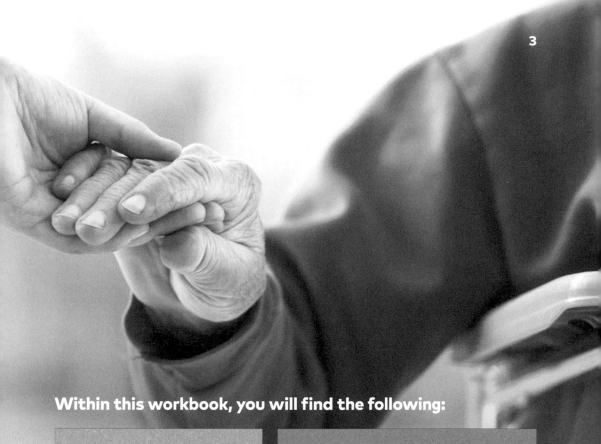

Within this workbook, you will find the following:

Tip sheets
These offer practical pointers for managing the complex issues that arise when you care for someone with Parkinson's.

The tip sheets can be found throughout this book with blue page borders.

Worksheets
These help you keep important information organized and easily located. Make copies or download more from **Parkinson.org/library**, so you can update them as information changes.

The worksheets can be found throughout this book with gray page borders.

Videos
Check out our CareMAP playlists at **Parkinson.org/videos** to watch videos with tips and advice from caregivers and care professionals to make your life easier.

Caregiver stories
You are not alone! Learn from and take comfort in the experiences of other people who care for someone with Parkinson's.

Contents

Resources

Contact the Parkinson's Foundation Helpline
Your first call can always be to the Parkinson's Foundation Helpline:
800-4PD-INFO (473-4636). Trained Parkinson's disease information
specialists will give you up-to-date information about Parkinson's, referrals
to healthcare professionals, a wide variety of free publications, emotional
support, community resources and more. You can also email us at
helpline@parkinson.org at any time.

AGING RESOURCES
These organizations offer information about services for all older adults.

Aging Life Care Association   520-881-8008, www.aginglifecare.org

National Association of Area Agencies on Aging   202-872-0888,
www.n4a.org

Alliance for Aging   800-96-ELDER (963-5337), www.allianceforaging.org

AARP   888-OUR-AARP (687-2277), www.aarp.org

Next Avenue   www.nextavenue.org
Read the special report, *Transforming Life as We Age*
www.nextavenue.org/special-section/transforming-life-age

CAREGIVER ASSOCIATIONS
These groups provide a range of options for caregiver education,
support and networking.

Family Caregiver Alliance   800-445-8106, www.caregiver.org

National Alliance for Caregiving   301-718-8444, www.caregiving.org

Caregiver Action Network   202-454-3970, www.caregiveraction.org

MEDICATION ASSISTANCE
There are general medication assistance programs as well as
programs specifically for low-income individuals and families.

NeedyMeds   800-503-6897, www.needymeds.org

Partnership for Prescription Assistance   www.pparx.org

Some pharmaceutical companies provide medication to people who
cannot afford it. **RxAssist** (www.rxassist.org) offers a database of
these patient assistance programs.

**Patient Access Network Foundation Parkinson's Disease
Assistance Program**   866-316-PANF (7263),
www.panfoundation.org/parkinsons-disease

There are various government programs you and the person with
Parkinson's might be eligible for. Call or visit their sites for information
and to find out whether you qualify.

Centers for Medicare and Medicaid Services
800-MEDICARE (800-633-4227), www.medicare.gov
Search or ask for the State Pharmaceutical Assistance Programs,
the Medicare Savings Programs and the free publication *Medicare & You.*

Social Security Administration   800-772-1213, www.ssa.gov
Search or ask for the Supplemental Security Income Benefits.

Eldercare Locator   800-677-1116, www.eldercare.gov

Department of Veterans Affairs   800-827-1000, www.va.gov

National Institute on Aging   800-222-2225, www.nia.nih.gov

ACTIVITIES OF DAILY LIVING
There are many products that can help with activities of daily living.
Below are just a few of the many companies that offer such products.

CLOTHING
Buck & Buck   800-458-0600, www.buckandbuck.com

MagnaReady   866-635-8866 www.magnaready.com

MEDICAL EQUIPMENT
Independent Living Aids, LLC   800-537-2118, www.independentliving.com

In-Step Mobility Products, Inc.   800-558-7837, www.ustep.com

National Seating and Mobility   615-595-1115, www.nsm-seating.com

Reliable Medical Supply, Inc.   763-255-3800, www.reliamed.com

ADVANCE DIRECTIVES
There are several groups that can help you document your medical
wishes and preferences.

American Bar Association   800-285-2221, www.americanbar.org
Search or ask for the Toolkit for Advance Planning.

Aging with Dignity, Five Wishes   www.agingwithdignity.org

National Hospice and Palliative Care Organization, Caring Connections
800-658-8898, www.caringinfo.org

**National Physician Orders for Life-Sustaining Treatment (POLST)
Organization**   503-494-4463, www.polst.org

My Contacts

Medical Contacts

PRIMARY CARE NAME: PHONE #:

ADDRESS: OTHER INFO:

NEUROLOGIST NAME: PHONE #:

ADDRESS: OTHER INFO:

DENTIST NAME: PHONE #:

ADDRESS: OTHER INFO:

EYE DOCTOR NAME: PHONE #:

ADDRESS: OTHER INFO:

PREFERRED HOSPITAL NAME: PHONE #:

ADDRESS: OTHER INFO:

PHARMACY NAME: PHONE #:

ADDRESS: OTHER INFO:

OTHER NAME: PHONE #:

ADDRESS: OTHER INFO:

OTHER NAME: PHONE #:

ADDRESS: OTHER INFO:

OTHER NAME: PHONE #:

ADDRESS: OTHER INFO:

Personal Contacts

EMERGENCY CONTACT NAME: PHONE #:

ADDRESS: OTHER INFO:

FRIEND/FAMILY NAME: PHONE #:

ADDRESS: OTHER INFO:

FRIEND/FAMILY NAME: PHONE #:

ADDRESS: OTHER INFO:

NEIGHBOR NAME: PHONE #:

ADDRESS: OTHER INFO:

TRANSPORTATION SERVICE NAME: PHONE #:

ADDRESS: OTHER INFO:

GROCERY HOME DELIVERY NAME: PHONE #:

ADDRESS: OTHER INFO:

OTHER NAME: PHONE #:

ADDRESS: OTHER INFO:

OTHER NAME: PHONE #:

ADDRESS: OTHER INFO:

OTHER NAME: PHONE #:

ADDRESS: OTHER INFO:

Acknowledgements

This book was written and reviewed by experts in Parkinson's disease and Parkinson's care:

Joan Gardner, RN, BSN
Rose Wichmann, PT
Struthers Parkinson's Center

Diane Breslow, MSW, LCSW

Paula Wiener, MSW, LCSW
Parkinson's Foundation

This book has been made possible through the generous donations of thousands of individuals affected by Parkinson's and grants from

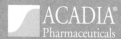

Design: Ultravirgo

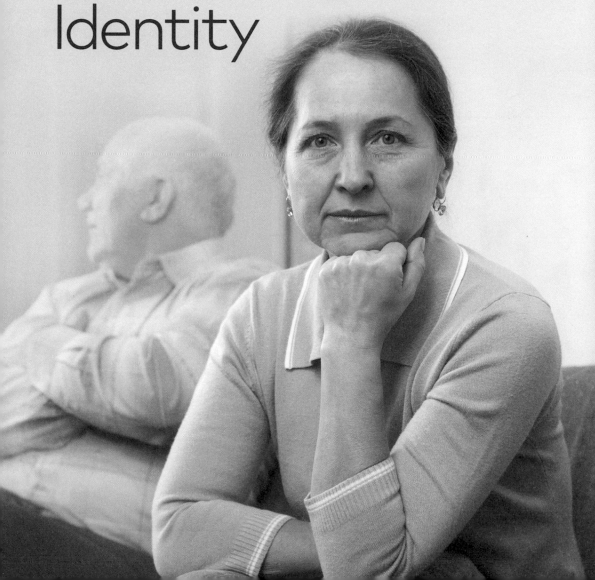

CHAPTER ONE

Early in the Journey: Your Caregiver Identity

Early in the Journey: Your Caregiver Identity

Parkinson's is a progressive disease: it changes over time. That can make it hard to define your role in your loved one's journey, as your involvement and responsibilities will change along the way. This section includes tip sheets related to figuring out how Parkinson's fits into your life. This includes sharing the diagnosis with family, assessing your work life and prioritizing your own needs.

IN THIS CHAPTER

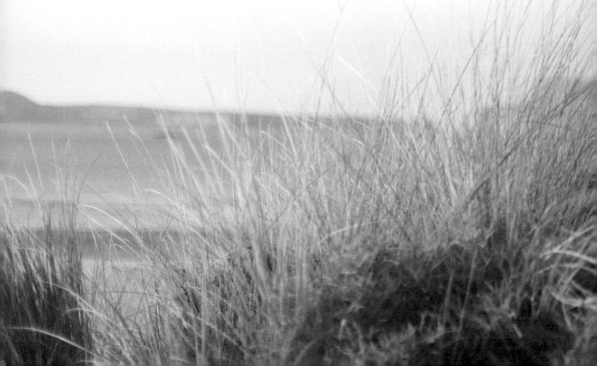

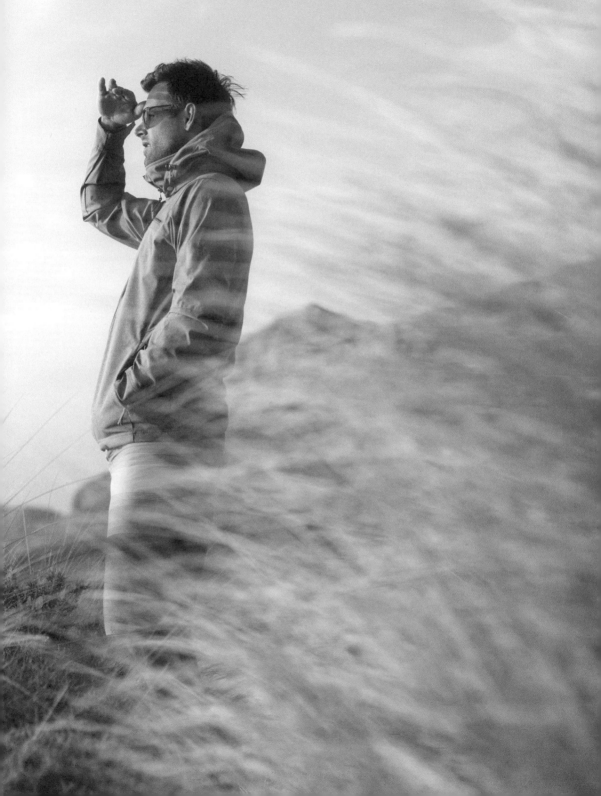

Caregiver Identity

While your loved one's Parkinson's diagnosis probably changed your life overnight, caregiver is a role and an identity that you grow into.

Each person with Parkinson's is unique, and so is each caregiver. As you start the journey, define "caregiving" for yourself. For some people, caregiver is one of many roles, or a group they belong to. For others, it is a central characteristic.

Many people do not like the term "caregiver." Especially early in the Parkinson's journey, you might not feel like you are actually "giving" care. Similarly, the person with Parkinson's might not see himself or herself as someone in need of care. But remember, care is not limited to physical tasks. Care can be emotional and spiritual as well as physical.

However you define it, and whatever term you choose – caregiver, care partner, carer, etc. – it is important that you accept this new role. It does not have to erase or replace any existing ways you self-identify; it is an addition, a new facet of your identity that will help you and your loved one face Parkinson's disease together.

As your loved one progresses through stages of Parkinson's, you will progress through stages of caring. You will have to take on new tasks and learn new skills. Learn all you can about the disease early on, so you can participate in healthcare discussions, make informed decisions and provide emotional and physical support now and as needed in the future. And always remember to consider your own needs for wellness, self-care and support.

How to Talk with Your Family About Parkinson's

Family members want to understand and help. How do you begin to explain Parkinson's disease to them?

First, you must understand the disease yourself. The Parkinson's Foundation offers several options to help you and your family learn all about Parkinson's disease (PD), including warning signs, diagnosis, symptoms, treatment, living well and much more.

» Explore **Parkinson.org** for information on any PD topic.

» Call our **toll-free Helpline at 1-800-4PD-INFO (473-4636)**. Our PD Information Specialists can answer your questions, provide resources and offer referrals and support.

» Order your free copy of our publication ***What You and Your Family Should Know***. Get it online (Parkinson.org/books) or by calling the Parkinson's Foundation Helpline.

Your family may have questions or fears about Parkinson's and genetics. For the vast majority of people, Parkinson's is not inherited. There is no test that can accurately predict who will develop Parkinson's. Extensive gene and biomarker research is underway to uncover the possible precursors – not necessarily causes – to disease development.

People unfamiliar with Parkinson's often think of it only as a disorder of movement. It is important to help family understand that there are other facets of the disease, and these can have an even greater impact on quality of life than the motor symptoms. Emphasize that Parkinson's is an ongoing journey, one in which we need to face realities little by little, make adaptations, stay connected to the people and things that are important to us and live each day in the best way possible.

Engage your family to help them understand.

» **Include your family in care planning discussions**. Ask for their observations about how the person with Parkinson's is doing.

» **Make specific, concrete requests** to your family members about how they can help you or the person with PD.

» **If your family members live out of town,** refer them to the Parkinson's Foundation website and Helpline for information, referrals and answers to any questions.

The 7 Needs of Caregivers

1 Education about Parkinson's disease

- **Understand the symptoms.**
- **Learn about available treatments.**
- **Consider the impact of Parkinson's on everyday life.**
- **Access resources.**
- **Explore your role in caregiving.**

2 Time management

- **Make daily and weekly lists of things to do.**
  Make sure the tasks are manageable and realistic.
- **Prioritize:** do the most important or difficult things first.
  Check off what's done.
- **Save up errands** to do more of them at one time.
- **Take a small task with you** if you are going some place
  where you have to wait.
- **Delegate what can be delegated.**
- **Forget unnecessary tasks.**
- **Take a break** when pressure gets too great, or as a reward.
- **Don't do so much in one area that you cannot be effective in another.**
- **Break large tasks into smaller, more doable parts.**
- **Establish and stick to routines.**
- **Recognize that some amount of time will be spent on things
  beyond your control.** Many tasks and activities will take longer
  for the person with Parkinson's as the disease progresses.

3 Self-care, health and respite

- **Build in quality time for yourself** (1–1½ hours a day, if possible) and protect it.
- **Keep up with your own needs, hobbies and regular activities.**
- **Exercise:** it leads to better sleep, decreased tension and depression and increased energy.
- **Eat a balanced, nutritious diet. Drink water.**
- **Recognize when you are stressed.**
- **Get enough rest.**
- **Take time to relax.**
- **Maintain a sense of humor.**
- **Get regular check-ups** and keep your own medical appointments.
- **Think about your future.**
  What goals do you hope to achieve, and how can you achieve them? Can your loved one help you achieve them?
- **Set limits and stick to them.**
  Bring in outside help (family or paid worker) so that you can take a break.

HOW TO CATEGORIZE AND PRIORITIZE NEEDS:
Building Your Plan

1. Identify your concerns according to the categories in this section.

2. Place your needs and concerns in priority order.

3. Consider and write down "action steps" that you can take.

4. Discuss your ideas with others.

5. Devise a step-by-step plan.

6. Implement the steps with help from others as needed.

4 A support team

- **Share the care.** Explore ways to get assistance and support as needed. This may include both physical and emotional help.

- **Develop your coping skills.** Caregivers experience a wide variety of emotions. Give yourself permission to feel sad or frustrated at times, but also take time to enjoy life. Focus on the present, the needs and rewards of the day. Try not to be critical of yourself in moments of anger. Give yourself credit, not guilt, and try to forgive any mistakes. Use positive self-talk: for example, tell yourself, "I am doing a good job." Know that it is okay to grieve the losses that you and your loved one may experience. Research shows that writing – in a journal or other format – can help you work through your feelings and emotions. What causes you to mourn? Where do you find satisfaction and pleasure?

- **Develop your emotional and spiritual support networks.** Include your healthcare team (physician, nurse, social worker, etc.), family, friends, neighbors, support group and individual support group members, clergy, volunteers and online support forums. Seek comfort from your faith, faith community and spiritual practices. Find meaning, insight, understanding and your own inner strengths. Adjust your expectations: Life and you are not perfect. Accept changes as they occur. Get help if necessary. Remember, it is a strength, not a weakness, to ask for help, including emotional help or counseling. Each person experiences depression in a unique way. It is important to take seriously any symptoms you experience that could signal depression; you should not feel embarrassed or ashamed.

- **Be aware of the core symptoms of depression:**
  - Sleeplessness
  - Loss of appetite
  - Difficulty concentrating
  - Feeling slowed down or restless inside
  - No interest in once-pleasurable activities
  - Thoughts of death or suicide
  - Feelings of hopelessness and worthlessness

If you think you may be depressed, talk to a doctor or mental health professional about your symptoms. Find a supportive professional that you trust and with whom you feel comfortable. In most cases, depression is effectively treated with psychotherapy, antidepressant medications or a combination of both, plus activities such as regular exercise, spirituality, supportive social interactions and meditation.

5 Your relationship with the person with Parkinson's

- **Maintain open communication.**
- **When conversing, remove or turn off loud and distracting noises.**
- **Express love and appreciation as well as concerns and feelings of frustration.** Don't let those feelings transform into resentments.
- **Match your expectations to the reality of your loved one's actions and abilities.**
- **Share special time together apart from caregiving tasks.**

6 Medical, financial and care decisions

- **Define and clarify issues,** including family participation in caregiving, advance directives, long-term care options or other topics as early us possible.
- **Devise steps for carrying out these plans.**
- When making decisions about hands-on care, **ask if your decision promotes your loved one's independence**: Do not confuse "caring" with "doing."

7 Community resources

- **Take advantage of physical and practical assistance and products.**
- **See what resources local associations have to offer.**
- **Seek education materials.** Many organizations (including the Parkinson's Foundation) provide these for free.
- Get **legal documents** (e.g., power of attorney for healthcare) in order. *(See "Planning Ahead" section starting on page 115 for more information.)*
- **Explore resources for financial assistance**, e.g., disability.
- **Reach out to a variety of professionals**, such as specialist physicians, nurses, therapists, social workers and clergy.

Balancing Work and Caregiving

Caring for someone with Parkinson's disease can be a full-time job, especially as the disease progresses to a more advanced stage. At first, you may be hesitant to tell your employer about your situation. However, it may be helpful to see if your workplace offers any special accommodations for caregivers.

- **Look into your company's personnel policies.** Check your employee handbook or staff website, or talk to someone from the human resources department to learn if your company offers programs or special assistance for caregivers. If you are a union member, ask a union representative to help you negotiate with your employer.

- **Arrange a meeting with your boss, and prepare for it in advance.** Before you approach your boss, decide if you want to discuss your situation as a caregiver, or if you want to go further and request specific job accommodations. Jot down the most important points you want to address.

- **Be upfront and positive.** When you meet with your supervisor, highlight your strengths and contributions to the company. Indicate your willingness to work together to identify potential accommodations to help you continue to do your job while maintaining your role as caregiver.

- **Get it in writing.** Send an email to your manager or HR representative with your understanding of the agreed-upon conditions. This will give everyone a reference point.

Later, if you consider leaving work altogether to accommodate your caregiving duties, consider the following steps:

- **Explore your options.** What are your alternatives to resigning? For example, can you take a career break or retire early? Will your employer let you work remotely or part-time? Would you want to consult or freelance on a schedule that is more suitable to your needs?

- **Take the time you need.** The Family Medical Leave Act (FMLA) entitles eligible employees of covered employers to take unpaid, job-protected leave for specified family and medical reasons. During such leave, group health insurance coverage continues under the same terms and conditions as before the leave. Eligible employees are entitled to 12 weeks of leave in a 12-month period in order to care for a spouse, child or parent with a serious health condition.

- **Understand the repercussions of your options.** Ask yourself: Can I manage with less money (and any effect on a pension or retirement plan)? Do not take this decision lightly. Think about the current and future loss of income if you leave your job. In addition to the possible financial consequences, you should consider the potential loss of independence, social contact and valuable skills. This may cause sadness or resentment. At the same time, the person with Parkinson's may feel bitter about his or her own loss of independence. Both of you must come to terms with these changes and these emotions.

I'm a writer, and I do have to spend a lot of time in my profession working, lecturing and giving workshops, and that's not easy to do. It is easy if you've taken out a long-term insurance policy and somebody comes every day and it's taken care of, otherwise it can be a big financial burden. I find that I just have to take time because it's our income and it's our livelihood. Jerry's very understanding about that.

– CAROLYN, CARES FOR HUSBAND, GERALD

It's a matter of waking up in the morning and saying, 'I'm glad I'm here, I'm going to make the best of it, and I really am going to enjoy my life.' Forget about Parkinson's; it's not going to go away. But we can deal with it, we can handle it and we can find wonderful things to do with our lives.

– CAROLYN, CARES FOR HUSBAND, GERALD

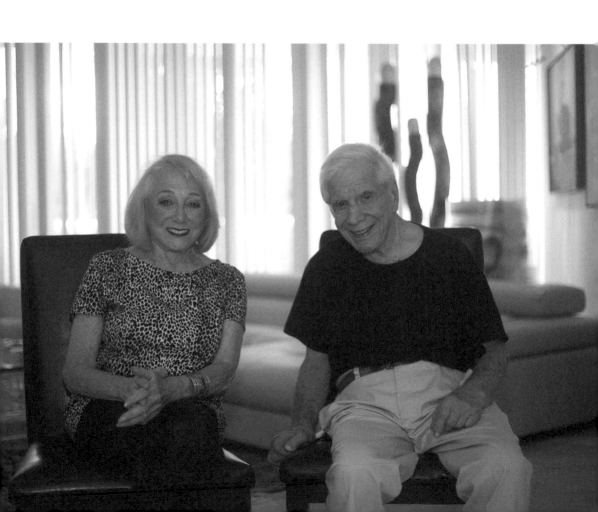

CHAPTER TWO

Caring for the Caregiver

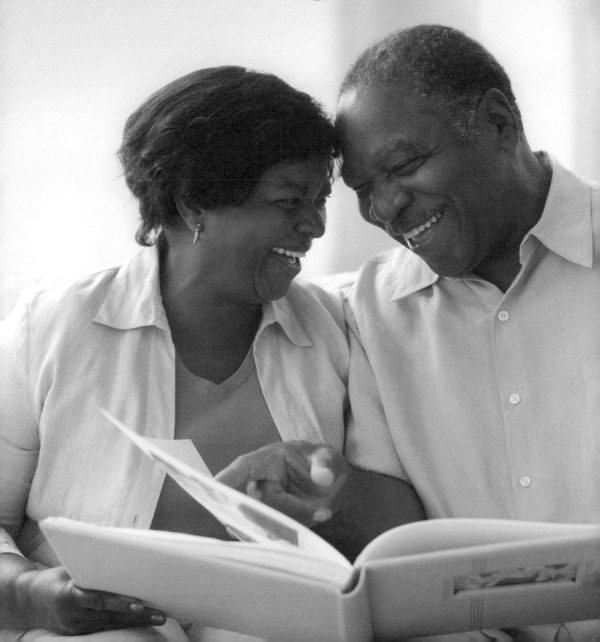

Caring for the Caregiver

Caregivers have an enormous, often underappreciated job. The job is unique for each caregiver but carries many common stresses, concerns, fears and rewards. This section is designed to help you, the caregiver, understand and handle your own particular caregiving situation, so the role can continue to be – or return to being – a healthy, viable, even rewarding option for you.

IN THIS CHAPTER

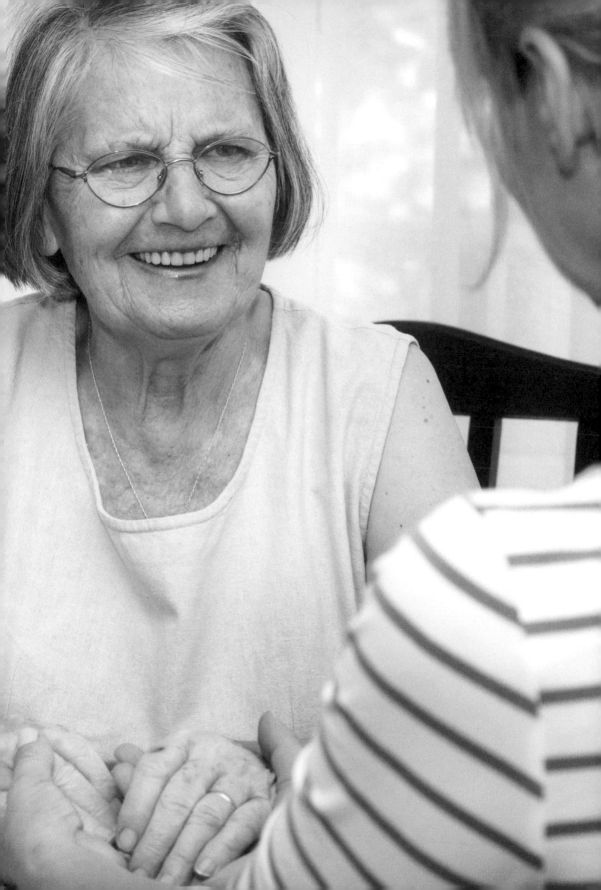

Caring for You

You may be involved in assisting the person with Parkinson's with many activities of daily living and medical tasks, as well as maintaining a household; shopping and preparing meals; organizing records, papers and appointments; transporting your loved one to healthcare visits; keeping up with social and family relationships and many other tasks. At the same time, you may be working, raising children or grandchildren or coping with your own health or personal issues.

Research from the National Alliance for Caregiving shows the top four caregiver concerns:

1) Keeping your loved one safe
2) Managing your own stress
3) Finding activities to do with your loved one
4) Taking time for yourself

Research also reveals that when caregivers are asked what they want, the majority respond that they want information about coping with being a caregiver. This information takes several forms, including knowledge about the disease, comfort with the caregiving role and managing stress. The following tips can help you cope.

» **Forgive yourself for not being perfect.** Caring for someone with a chronic illness means your world has been turned upside down. Your daily routine will definitely change, and you will probably have to compromise some of your personal standards of housekeeping, meal preparation and other tasks. Accept your own humanity. Give yourself a pat on the back for doing the best you can.

WATCH THE VIDEO

Advice for Caregivers, from Caregivers

Online at Parkinson.org/videos in the "CareMAP Caregiver Stories" playlist

» **Acknowledge your right to feel emotionally off-balance.** Recognize the hidden grief component of your anger, anxiety, guilt and depression. Expect adaptation to, but not resolution of, your grief. Accept it and seek out someone who understands it.

» **Determine your limits.** What is your comfort level providing care? Some people feel uncomfortable when incontinence becomes an issue. Some determine they can provide care at home as long as others in the family can put up with the disruptions. Everyone has limits. What are yours?

» **Make regular breaks from caregiving a priority.** You cannot be a good caregiver to someone else if you do not take care of yourself. Your loved one can survive a few hours and, periodically, a few days without you.

» **Be kind to yourself.** Remember you are experiencing normal reactions to abnormal circumstances.

» **Seek out joy in your relationship with the person with Parkinson's.** Your hands-on duties, such as bathing and dressing your loved one, might feel like work, but these tasks bring you together. Add some fun to your hands-on care: sing songs, tell jokes, share goals and dreams.

» **Develop a habit of participating in activities together outside cares.** Shared time as husband-wife, mother-daughter, siblings or other relationship – rather than as caregiver and care recipient, or even care partners – allows you to enjoy each other and build happy memories.

» **Try to forgive your loved one for past hurts.** Resentment toward past wrongs and injustices will make your present caregiving role difficult. Let go of what was, and concentrate on making what is healthy and productive.

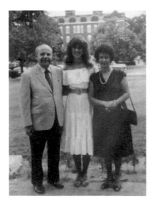

Being a caregiver is probably the most difficult job you're ever going to have. The only way you can do it is to take care of yourself. You cannot say, 'I don't have time for me.' The person you're taking care of wants the best for you because you're giving the best to them. Don't be a martyr. It's okay to take care of yourself.

– KAREN, CARED FOR FATHER, JOSEPH

Finding Meaning in Caregiving

Like most things in life, caregiving is not an either/or experience. Caregiving offers trials and triumphs as well as challenges and joys. A *Caring Today* survey found that a majority of caregivers experience the role as "more rewarding than expected." This is significant information: If the Parkinson's community – professionals as well as those personally affected by PD – can help people through the hurdles, they can potentially find more positives in the experience.

What are some caregiver rewards?

Connection: Few people plan ahead for the role of caregiver. At first, you may think you are alone. You will probably figure out that there are many others in the same situation. You make friends. You adopt an identity as "caregiver" (or care partner, or carer). You discover new interests and endeavors.

Relationships: Accept and be thankful for the help of family and friends, and appreciate your quality time with them. Although "sharing the care" can sometimes lead to conflict, people who have worked through this with some success find that it can actually bring families closer. In addition, your caregiving role might bring a feeling of increased closeness to the person with Parkinson's.

Growth: Take pride in how much you have learned and in discovering your own strengths. Through caregiving you are likely to gain new insights about life. Find positives in every day, feel empowered and recognize your accomplishments.

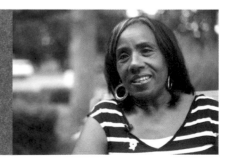

WATCH THE VIDEO

Caregiver Rewards and Challenges

Online at Parkinson.org/videos in the "CareMAP Caregiver Stories" playlist

The rewards are not limited to those on the previous page.
You may also experience the following, and many others:

- **Taking pleasure in giving**
  "I feel good that I am able to return the favor and take care of her."

- **Seeing positives**
  "I am grateful that I have my health."

- **Exploring new spiritual beliefs or revisiting old ones**
  "My beliefs and faith keep me going."

- **Feeling proud and purposeful**
  "I am doing what's right and fulfilling my responsibility."

Benefits of Support Groups
- Commonality among members
- Education, information
- Learning to adjust to diagnosis
- Practical techniques
- Feeling understood
- Reducing stigma
- Socialization and friendships

*In 2016, the Parkinson's Foundation hosted a Caregiver Summit that brought together care partners from all over the world to share experiences and everyday strategies for caring for a person with Parkinson's and caring for yourself. Watch the presentations in the "Caregiver Summit 2016" playlist at **Parkinson.org/videos**.*

When you go to the support groups, when you go to the meetings, you meet other people with the same problems, the same difficulties. It's a wonderful way to communicate, understand what you're up against and get advice from other people. As you get together you start talking, you start confiding, and you find that you get people that are very willing to listen. That's very important to me.

– CAROLYN, CARES FOR HUSBAND, GERALD

CARING MOMENT

Take regular "me time."

Whether it's for an hour, a day or a week, make yourself a priority on a regular basis, and do not feel guilty about it.

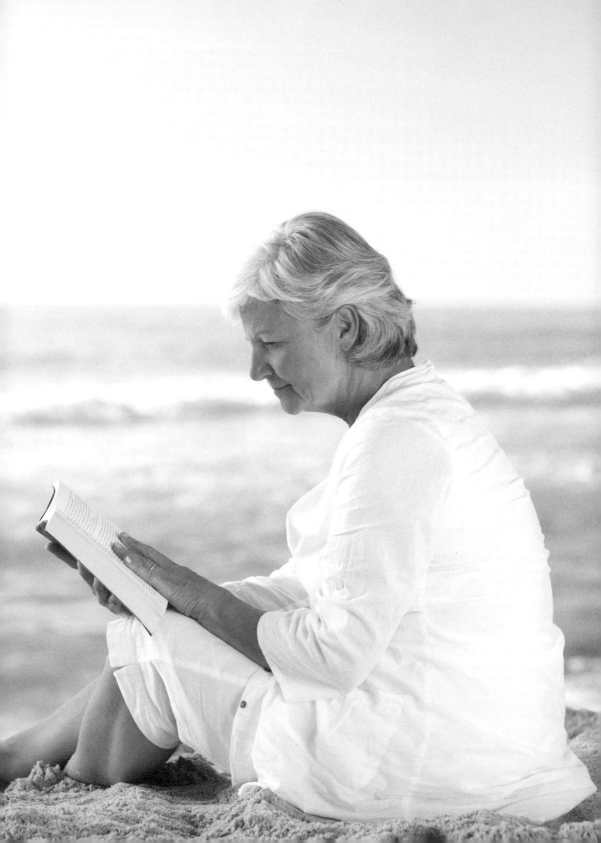

Managing Caregiver Stress

Some health professionals call caregivers "hidden patients."
You need emotional support and practical services just
like people with Parkinson's. With all your responsibilities
related to maintaining a home, family and career in addition
to caring, stress is an inevitability. Long-term family
caregivers often find it challenging to reduce stressors.
Here are some techniques to help you manage stress.

Active Stress Reduction

» **Exercise away the anxiety.** Talk to your doctor or physical therapist
about setting up an exercise regimen that meets your health needs.

» **Exercise with others.** This simultaneously meets two important needs:
exercise and social support.

» **Socialize with people who uplift you.** Nothing can empower you like a
feeling of camaraderie. Minimize exposure to negative people. Instead,
go out with friends or get involved with a community organization,
support group or charity that you believe in.

» **Learn to laugh.** Keeping a sense of humor helps beat anxiety.
Watch a funny video or read something funny every day.

Breathing Awareness

» **Create a relaxing space** that will minimize interruptions and distractions.
  – Turn down/off your telephones.
  – Dim the lighting in the room.

» **Sit or lie down with your body supported.**

» **Close your eyes and focus your attention on your breathing.**

» **Inhale through the nose.**
  – Feel abdomen expand first, then ribcage, then chest.
  – Exhale long and slow in reverse order.

» **Keep breath rhythmic**; don't force or hold breath.

Practice for 5–10 minutes daily. Use this technique whenever you feel stress
or loss of control over your body or emotions.

Body Awareness

» As you practice deep breathing, **mentally identify areas of your body** starting from the head.

» **"Listening" to your body's signals** allows you to focus your attention on specific areas of muscle tension. **Release the tension**; feel your body "sink" into the support beneath you.

» **Make sure your position is balanced** with equal weight on both sides of the body, stretched out, open and extended. Try lying on your back, arms at sides, legs slightly apart; bend knees if that is more comfortable.

Progressive Muscle Relaxation Technique

This relaxation exercise involves tightening each muscle group in your body, holding for 5 seconds, and then gradually releasing and relaxing for 10-15 seconds. It takes about 20 minutes to perform and can bring tremendous benefits if you fit it into your daily routine.

1. Sit or lie down quietly in a comfortable position, with no distractions or possibilities of interruption. Begin by thinking slow, relaxing thoughts. Bring to mind any comfortable image you can imagine, such as lying by a stream in a beautiful forest. Take three deep breaths and focus on the tension in your body.

2. Go through each of the muscle groups, beginning with the hands, working up to the body then down to the feet. With practice you will soon be familiar with the sequence. Tense the muscles as tightly as you can. Hold for 5 seconds, then gradually release.

3. As you release the muscles, relax and feel the tension drain away. Imagine the blood circulating in the different muscle groups. Concentrate on the feelings in the muscles as they go from tight to loose. Notice the difference between tension and relaxation. Perform the tightening and relaxing of each muscle group twice before moving on.

Recommended Relaxation Recordings
Script and music: Nielsen/Miller/Holton: "Healing Blue Sky," Bernie Siegel, Janalea Hoffman

Environmental: "Solitudes" series, Natural Sound Series

Piano: David Lanz, Danny Wright, Michael Jones

Guitar: Will Ackerman

Bamboo/Native American Flute: R. Carlos Nakai, Richard Warner, Christian Nielsen

Harp: Kim Robertson, Joel Andrews, Hilary Stagg

Classical: Adagio collection, Lind Institute collection

Religious: Jon Simon (Jewish), Mary Beth Carlson, Lorie Line, John Michael Talbot (Christian), Benedictine Monks (Gregorian Chant)

DID YOU KNOW?
According to the *Parkinson's Outcomes Project*, the largest clinical study of Parkinson's ever conducted, a change in caregiver can negatively impact the health of both the person with Parkinson's and the new caregiver. For the person with Parkinson's, the transition is associated with worsening clinical outcomes and health-related quality of life. For the incoming caregiver, particularly family members newly introduced to Parkinson's care, caregiver strain is a serious concern.

Ultimately, finding balance in your mind and body will help you cope with the daily stresses of life. This may mean limiting your exposure to environmental stressors or using complementary therapies. Such approaches are wonderful ways to lower anxiety, lower blood pressure and improve your well-being.

if you feel that you are totally overwhelmed by your feelings, consult with your physician. He or she can refer you to a mental health professional. There is no shame in seeking help when you need it.

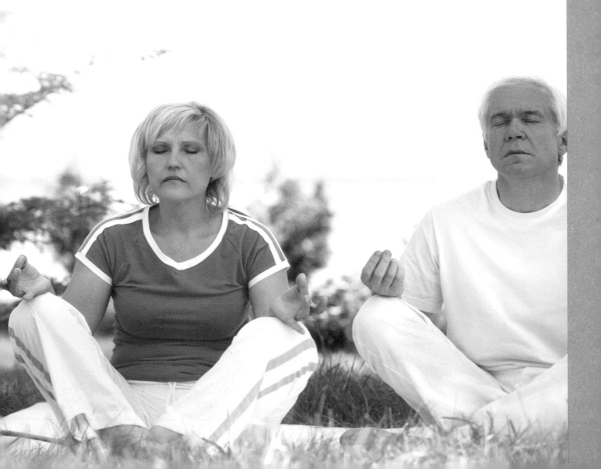

CHECKLIST FOR BUILDING GOOD SLEEP HABITS

☐ Establish a regular bedtime and morning awakening time that you maintain seven days per week.

☐ Design and maintain a comforting bedtime ritual.

☐ Turn off the television.

☐ If weaning yourself from bedtime television is difficult, try substituting relaxing music.

☐ Customize your sleep environment; invest in a good mattress and pillow.

☐ Keep noise and light levels low.

☐ Maintain a slightly cool room temperature.

☐ Keep pets from your bed.

☐ Designate your bedroom for sleep and sex; it is not an all-purpose space.

☐ Avoid strenuous exercise, alcohol, nicotine and caffeine within four hours of your bedtime.

☐ Eliminate "checking the clock" throughout the night.

☐ Limit prescription sedatives to a two-week period.

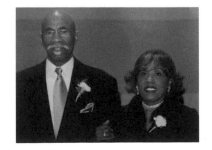

As long as you dress up, with makeup on and your hair done, they think you're okay. And some days I'm crushed.

– RUTH, CARES FOR HUSBAND, HENRY

CHAPTER TWO: CARING FOR THE CAREGIVER

Worksheet

Caregiver Self-Assessment

Perform this self-assessment at regular intervals to identify your risk factors and shed light on your needs. There is great value in assessing yourself:

• Become more self-aware now and over time.

• Measure your reactions to various aspects of caregiving.

• Tease out the areas of greatest concern to you.

• Acknowledge and validate your role, experiences and feelings.

• Put into words an experience that you may have been unable to define, e.g., "How do I balance my needs with the needs of my partner?"

Share the results of your self-assessment with family, friends or others close to you so they can better understand the scope of caregiving (emotional, physical, fiscal, social). This might lead them to become more engaged in caring for the person with Parkinson's or support you in other ways.

FILLED OUT BY: DATE:

Rate each item below from 1 (almost always) to 5 (never) according to how much of the time each statement applies to you. Write the date above so you can track your wellbeing over time.

1 = ALMOST ALWAYS
2 = FREQUENTLY
3 = OCCASIONALLY
4 = RARELY
5 = NEVER

1. I exercise on a regular basis.   1 2 3 4 5

2. I make and keep preventive and necessary medical and dental appointments.   1 2 3 4 5

3. I have a job or regular volunteer activity that is gratifying.   1 2 3 4 5

4. I do not use tobacco products.   1 2 3 4 5

5. I do not use alcohol or drugs.   1 2 3 4 5

6. I get an adequate amount of sleep each day.   1 2 3 4 5

7. I have a hobby or recreational activity I enjoy and spend time doing.   1 2 3 4 5

8. I eat at least two to three balanced meals a day.   1 2 3 4 5

9. I have at least one person in whom I can confide (tell my problems, discuss my successes).   1 2 3 4 5

10. I take time to do things that are important to me (e.g., church, garden, read, spend time alone).   1 2 3 4 5

11. I do not have problems with sleeplessness or anxiety.   1 2 3 4 5

12. I have personal goals and am taking steps to achieve them.   1 2 3 4 5

TOTAL SCORE:
Add the numbers, and compare to the scale on the next page

INTERPRETATION:

12–24   You are doing an excellent job taking care of yourself.

25–36   You have room for improvement. Examine the areas where you struggle, and seek help from family, friends or healthcare professionals to make some changes.

37–48   You are doing a poor job taking care of yourself and are at moderate risk for personal health problems. Talk to your healthcare provider or others who can help you create and stick to a plan to take better care of yourself.

48–60   You are at extremely high risk for personal health problems. It is important for you to talk to your personal healthcare provider as soon as possible. Remember, you can only provide good care for someone else if you take good care of yourself.

Adapted from "Checklist for Caregivers: Do You Take Care of Yourself?" Bass, D.S. 1990, *Caring Families: Supports and Interventions*, p. 35, National Association of Social Workers.

CHAPTER THREE

Practical Pointers

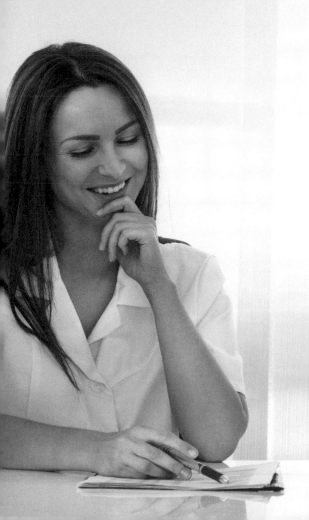
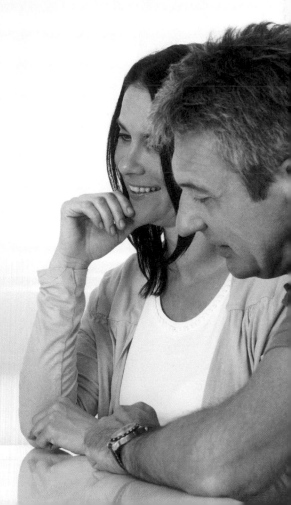

Practical Pointers

Parkinson's can be full of surprises. As a caregiver, it takes skill and patience to know when to assist with a task and when to simply allow the person more time to do the task independently. This section contains tips and strategies you can use to make the most of each day.

IN THIS CHAPTER

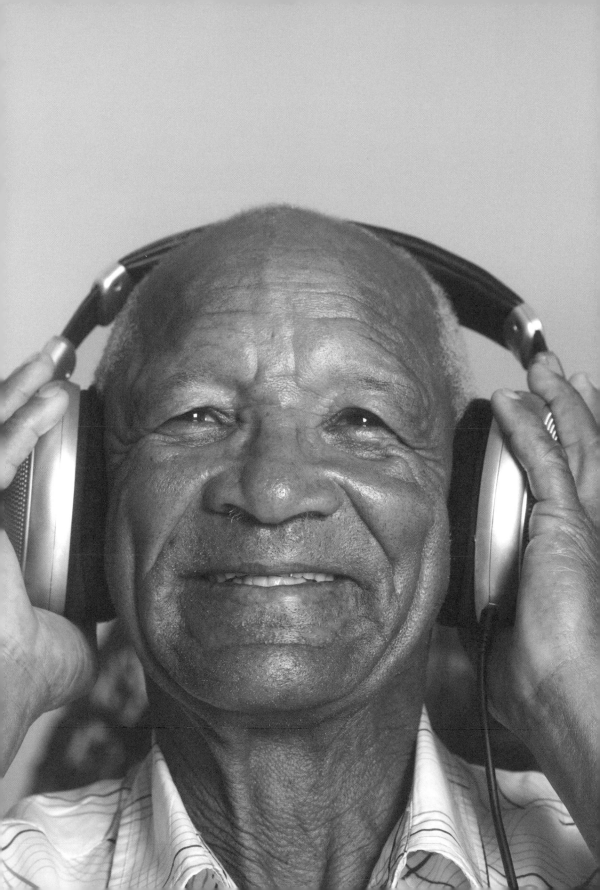

Organizing Medical Information

The incidence and severity of Parkinson's symptoms vary from day to day, even from one time of day to another. Being organized and planning for many potential outcomes can help you put a positive spin on what might otherwise be a stressful situation.

Keep an organized record of your loved one's medical and surgical history. This will come in handy when the person with Parkinson's needs to fill out forms and answer questions about his or her health history. Use a notebook or three-ringed binder to write the medical and surgical history, so new information can easily be added. If you choose to keep records electronically, make sure you have a way to access it when you go to appointments, or keep a separate hard copy to bring with you.

Keep all of the following information in the notebook or binder:

- **Healthcare directive:** Create this document with the person with Parkinson's, with input from the family and the healthcare team. Give copies to your loved one's physicians, and keep a copy in the binder.
- **Names, addresses and phone numbers** of your loved one's primary care doctor and other medical specialists
- **Up-to-date medication list**: List each medication with strengths and times. For example: carbidopa/levodopa 25/100, 1 pill four times a day – 8am, 12pm, 4pm, 8pm. The medication list can be kept on the computer (and printed for the binder) or written down. Either way, it must be updated after every medication change.
- **Clinic visit notes**
- **Appointment schedules**

It's really helpful if there is a care partner who can help to listen during appointments, talk about the questions and jot the things down – especially if you lose your handwriting.

– LYLE, CARES FOR WIFE, LAVON

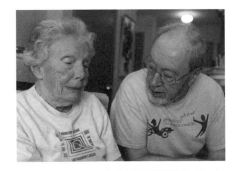

Communicating with the Healthcare Team

Open, honest communication between you, your loved one and the healthcare team is crucial. While you depend on health professionals for high quality care, they depend on you for information about the patient's health status and living experience, and for properly carrying out professional advice.

So, who is on the healthcare team? The primary care physician will likely be your main point of contact, but there are many specialists who can participate in your loved one's care:

- Neurologist (preferably a movement disorders specialist – a neurologist with special training in movement disorders)
- Nurse practitioner or physician assistant
- Nurse
- Pharmacist
- Physical therapist
- Occupational therapist
- Speech-language pathologist
- Social worker
- Registered dietician
- Psychologist or psychiatrist

If your loved one has an appointment with a healthcare provider who does not specialize in Parkinson's disease or movement disorders, help that person provide high quality PD care by telling him or her about professional education opportunities from the Parkinson's Foundation. Our online courses, webinars and Allied Team Training for Parkinson's program will teach healthcare providers best practices in Parkinson's team care and help them make more informed treatment decisions for their patients with PD. They can learn more at **Parkinson.org/professionaleducation**.

The only predictable thing about this disease is that it is unpredictable.

– RICHARD, DIAGNOSED AT 36

Go to All the Medical Appointments

Be present at every appointment with the person with Parkinson's. **You are there to be supportive and take notes, but also to ask questions and share information.** Your ability to communicate with healthcare providers can influence the quality of care your loved one receives. In fact, some movement disorders specialists insist that a caregiver be in the room for every visit. As patients, regardless of our ailment, we often say we are doing "fine," even when that is not the whole truth. As a caregiver, you can provide specific information on problems the person with Parkinson's is having. This can help the doctor make necessary adjustments to the treatment regimen.

At the same time, it is important to make sure that the person with Parkinson's feels empowered in conversations with all healthcare providers. After all, you are talking about his care. If your loved one is able to speak for himself, encourage him to share any changes or concerns with the doctor. Then add your own observations.

Both you and the person with Parkinson's should be honest and ask direct questions. If something is wrong, the provider should say so, but it helps to ask. If you have doubts, get a second opinion. Even the experts do not always agree about the best treatment.

Remember, healthcare providers see many patients in a day and only see your loved one with PD briefly in the office. You are with him all the time. Therefore, it is important that you know all about your loved one's medical conditions (PD and others), including medications and other treatments, so you can make the most of your time with the provider. Go to each appointment with a written list of questions that you want to cover as well as problems or improvements that may have arisen since the last visit. Prioritize your questions; sometimes the appointment schedule does not allow you to ask everything on your list. If you cannot get all your questions answered at the visit, ask your doctor or staff at the clinic who you can contact with unanswered questions or new concerns.

DID YOU KNOW? ....

The Parkinson's Foundation's *Parkinson's Outcomes Project*, the largest-ever clinical study of Parkinson's, found that depression and anxiety are the number one factors impacting the overall health status of people with PD. Make sure a doctor screens your loved one for depression at least once a year.

Being at the appointment is also important because of rules about privacy and confidentiality (you might have heard of HIPAA, the Health Insurance Portability and Accountability Act). Unless you are physically in the room with the patient and the doctor, the doctor cannot give you information about your loved one's health and treatment just because you are related to the patient, even if you are the spouse.

Involve the Team

The team of doctors, nurses, rehab therapists and social workers can help your loved one live well with Parkinson's. Learn each team member's role and understand how to access their services when needed. Ask questions and state your concerns to help each team member meet your loved one's needs.

These individuals can teach you how to provide proper care for the person with Parkinson's. As the disease and symptoms progress, this will become particularly important. If the person with Parkinson's is hospitalized or receives therapy at a rehab facility, ask the staff to show you proper caregiving techniques for tasks like lifting, transfers and bathing. Learning basic skills will build your confidence in the role of physical caregiving.

Communicating with the Healthcare Team in the Hospital

Three out of four people with Parkinson's do not receive their medications on time when staying in the hospital. This can result in complications and a longer hospital stay. Be ready in the event of a planned or unplanned hospital stay by ordering a Parkinson's Foundation *Aware in Care* kit: call our Helpline at 1-800-4PD-INFO (473-4636) or order online at **Parkinson.org/store**. Review the materials when you receive the kit, so you will be ready to advocate for the person with Parkinson's when he or she is in the hospital.

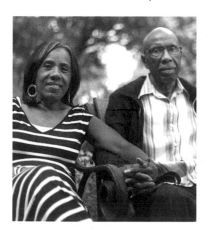

His doctor would look at me instead of talking to Henry. So I told him, 'You're supposed to talk to him, not me.' I was feeling that they thought he was less than. His voice gets low and it takes him a while to respond, but still give him the respect and show him the dignity to talk to him. It's his appointment, not mine.

– RUTH, CARES FOR HUSBAND, HENRY

Spend time together, apart from caregiving tasks.

A local outing or a trip down memory lane can add joy to your day and help reduce anxiety.

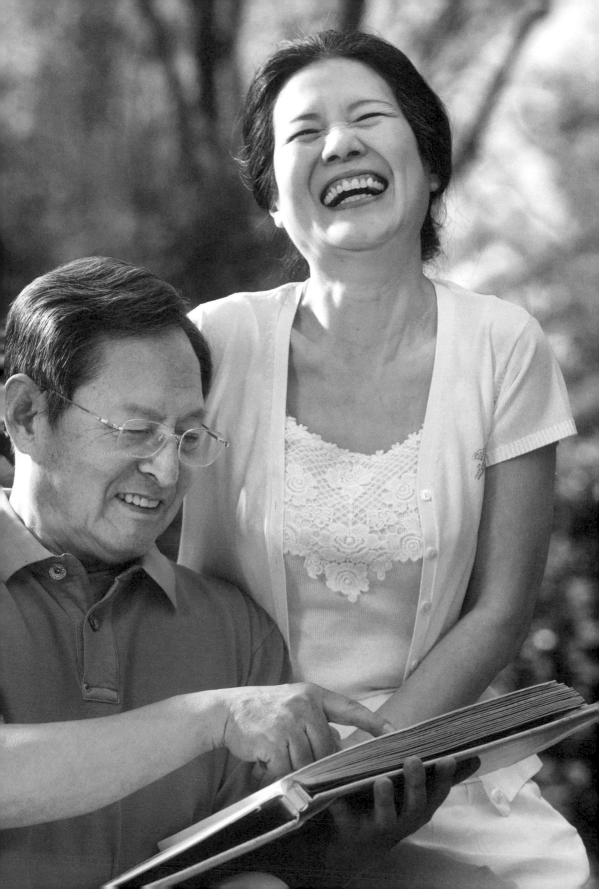

Preparing for a Medical Appointment

BEFORE THE APPOINTMENT

» **Schedule the appointment at a time that works well for everyone involved.**

» **Fill out the Medical Appointment Worksheet** on page 62.

» **The medical team will be better able to care for the person with Parkinson's if you are prepared for the appointment.** Think about (and write down) specific concerns you want to discuss with the doctor:

– Bothersome motor symptoms, such as tremor, slowness, stiffness, balance/falls

– Bothersome non-motor symptoms, such as mood, thinking changes, dizziness, sleep, constipation or pain

» **List any medical changes since the last appointment.** Was there a hospitalization or emergency room visit? Was there a surgery or procedure?

» If your loved one has had deep brain stimulation (DBS) surgery for Parkinson's, **is programming or a battery analysis needed**? This may require a separate appointment with a DBS programmer.

» If your loved one has had changes in walking, ability to complete day-to-day cares and activities, voice volume or swallowing, **an appointment with a rehab therapist** (physical, occupational or speech therapist) may be needed.

– If your clinic has rehab therapists on-site, call the doctor's office to see if a therapy appointment can be made for the same day as the medical appointment.

– If there is no rehab therapist on-site, you will need a referral for insurance coverage. Add this to your list of topics to bring up with the doctor.

» **Do you have questions about which exercise program is right for the person with Parkinson's?** Ask for a referral to a physical therapist who can tailor an exercise program for the person with Parkinson's.

» **Note any changes to the living situation.**

» **Check prescription bottles for needed refills.**

THE DAY BEFORE AND DAY OF THE APPOINTMENT

» **Assemble the following items to bring to the appointment:**

– Current medication list; include all prescription and over-the-counter medications and supplements (including strengths and doses)

– Insurance cards and ID

– Pill box (so medications can be given while away from home)

» If you want a letter from the visit to go to your loved one's primary doctor, **bring the name and address of the doctor** and clinic.

» **Plan to attend the appointment with your loved one.** It is helpful to have another person present to share observations, hear and understand the information discussed and take notes.

» **Get to the appointment on time, even early.** Make sure there is enough time to visit the restroom before the appointment.

DURING THE APPOINTMENT

» **Write notes and answers to questions.**

» **Be honest when answering questions**, even if the answers are difficult.

» **Understand the recommendations** and follow-up plans before you leave. If something is unclear, ask the doctor for clarification.

» **Make sure you get information about any new medications** that are prescribed:

– What is the name of the medication?

– What is the medication being prescribed for? Is it to replace another medication or to be taken in addition to other medications?

– What is the dose, and how often is it to be taken? (Many anti-Parkinson medications are increased gradually to avoid side effects. Make sure you write down the dosing schedule precisely.)

– When and how will you know if the medicine is working?

– Are there common or serious side effects to watch for?

» **Understand who you should call with questions, concerns or updates.**

» **Try to schedule the next appointment** or additional team appointments before leaving the office.

General Health

People with Parkinson's may have other health conditions, too, and they all require regular medical management. Your loved one may get a cold or the flu; develop a bladder infection; or be diagnosed with arthritis, diabetes, a heart or lung condition, cancer or other ailment. Be proactive in caring for all health concerns, not just Parkinson's.

It is important to remember that Parkinson's symptoms tend to change slowly over time. Sudden changes may signal a medical problem such as an infection. Emotional stress, worry and anxiety can also worsen PD symptoms. The neurologist may direct you to your loved one's primary care doctor for evaluation of a sudden change in symptoms.

Medical Information to Consider

- **Parkinson's disease medications often cause dry mouth**, which can result in dental problems. Make sure your loved one gets dental check-ups twice a year.
- Although there is no one special diet for people living with Parkinson's, your loved one should follow these general recommendations:
  - Drink 48-64 ounces of fluid daily.
  - Eat foods high in fiber. Choose fresh or frozen fruits and vegetables as well as whole grain pasta and bread.
- **Protein in foods can interfere with levodopa absorption.** Talk to the healthcare team about medication timing and meals.
- **Parkinson's can cause changes in blood pressure** that result in dizziness when you stand up. Tell the doctor if the person with Parkinson's experiences dizziness when standing up. The doctor should test for a condition called orthostatic hypotension by measuring blood pressure in both sitting and standing positions.
- **The person with Parkinson's should wear sunscreen when outside.** Point out any changes in the skin to a doctor.
- **Your loved one may develop dry or flaking skin on the face.** Use mild soap, warm water and creams, which are more moisturizing than lotions on the face.
- **The scalp may also become itchy and dry.** Try a shampoo containing selenium sulfide, salicylic acid, zinc or coal tar. Make sure you rinse shampoo thoroughly from hair. Switch products periodically. See a dermatologist if skin problems do not go away.

The Importance of Exercise and Activity for People with Parkinson's

People with Parkinson's who start exercising earlier experience a significant slower decline in quality of life than those who start later. Regular exercise can help combat muscle stiffness, posture changes and weakness; reduce balance, walking and other mobility changes; and manage constipation, which is commonly seen in people with PD.

You can encourage regular exercise and activity in the following ways:

» **Help your loved one establish a regular exercise routine.** Offer to join the person with Parkinson's for a walk, bike ride or visit to the local health club.

» **Allow the person with Parkinson's to be as independent as possible**, but help when needed. Certain tasks may now take longer to perform, and PD symptoms can change throughout the day.

» Loss of automatic movements can make the person with Parkinson's less inclined to move around, so **remind your loved one to change position at least every hour during the day**. People with Parkinson's should avoid long periods of time sitting. Suggest listening to an audiobook while walking around or try watching TV from a treadmill.

» **Encourage your loved one to pursue hobbies and activities.** Parkinson's disease can cause apathy or loss of motivation, and changes in motor control can make activities your loved one enjoyed in the past more difficult, so he or she may be less likely to participate without encouragement from others.

» **Seek a referral to a physical therapist** who can provide individual evaluation, recommend an exercise program and help with follow-through.

DID YOU KNOW?

Based on findings from the Parkinson's Foundation's *Parkinson's Outcomes Project*, the largest-ever clinical study of Parkinson's, it is recommended that people with PD engage in at least 2.5 hours of exercise a week for a better quality of life. Help your loved one get up and get moving! Visit Parkinson.org/exercise for more tips.

Cueing Strategies

Parkinson's disease impacts the ability to perform movements that are usually done without conscious thought.

As the disease progresses, your loved one's movements will become smaller and less automatic. Parkinson's can also result in inaccurate perception of movement size and quality, so your loved one may not fully recognize these changes. You can use cues to help your loved one move more easily. Simple cues can make the brain less dependent on its automatic systems and "reroute" messages so movement improves.

- **Keep it short.** Long explanations or instructions are often harder to follow for someone with Parkinson's disease. Use these simple phrases to cue movement:
    - "Stand tall" if posture becomes too flexed
    - "Big steps" to decrease shuffling when walking
    - "March" when turning to keep knees high

- Since Parkinson's impacts automatic movements, standing tall and taking big steps, for example, may not happen automatically. You will likely need to **repeat cues on a regular basis**.

Ask the doctor for a referral to a physical therapist who can tailor cueing strategies to your loved one's individual needs. In particular, there are many ways to help with walking challenges, such as freezing episodes.

Addressing Communication Challenges

Parkinson's disease can impact communication in many ways.

Most people with Parkinson's experience a soft voice volume and may be difficult to hear. Loss of automatic facial expression can be misinterpreted as boredom, anger or sadness. Mood changes in Parkinson's such as apathy, depression or anxiety can also affect communication. The following tips can make communication easier.

» **Try to have conversations one-on-one or in small groups.** Smaller groups will be more willing to pause the conversation and wait for a comment than a large group.

» **Reduce or remove distractions** like TV, radio or music when speaking to the person with Parkinson's.

» **Be close to each other when you talk** so it is easier to hear. Avoid yelling from another room in the house!

» **Encourage the person with Parkinson's to take a deep breath** before beginning to speak to enhance his or her vocal loudness.

» **Give the person with Parkinson's time to respond or participate in conversation.** Just like slowness in movement, thought processes can be slowed by Parkinson's disease.

» **Do not make assumptions about how your loved one is feeling based on facial expression.** Remember, you can't judge a book by its cover!

» **Recognize that mood changes such as depression, anxiety and apathy can be symptoms of Parkinson's disease.** If you notice these symptoms in your loved one, speak to his or her physician.

» **Seek a referral to a speech pathologist** who is certified in the Lee Silverman Voice Treatment therapy (visit www.lsvtglobal.com) or who has attended a Parkinson's Foundation Allied Team Training for Parkinson's program.

Coping with Fatigue

Many people with Parkinson's experience excessive daytime sleepiness. They report a loss of energy and chronic fatigue, which may be disruptive to planned activities and schedules.

Consider the following:

» **People with excessive daytime sleepiness (EDS) feel fatigue during the day and then have poor quality sleep at night.** Activities that make you tired may be bad for the morning, but excellent at night. Adding exercise to the routine may improve nighttime sleep quality.

» **Think about scheduling fewer activities each day.** The person with Parkinson's may have low energy and therefore may not be able to do as much as he or she used to do.

» **Consider breaking up tasks, errands or other activities into shorter time periods**, allowing for rest breaks as needed.

» **Schedule brief rest periods or naps** to restore your loved one's energy during the day. Be mindful that excessive daytime sleep may prevent someone from resting well at night.

» **Recognize that your schedule may need to be flexible** and responsive to how the person with Parkinson's is feeling. You may need to postpone or cancel activities based on these variations.

» **Have a back-up plan** in case the scheduled activity falls through.

» **Make sure travel schedules include enough time to accommodate rest periods.**

» **Be aware that the person with Parkinson's may request more assistance when feeling fatigued.** Offer help as needed.

» **Encourage your loved one to avoid tasks that require significant coordination or attention when fatigued** to avoid accidents or falls.

Making Daily Life Easier

Even simple, routine tasks can become more challenging as Parkinson's disease progresses.

The following changes can make home tasks easier to perform:

» **Relocate frequently used items** in the kitchen, bedroom and bathroom to a place where they can be readily accessed by your loved one.

» **Label drawers and cabinets** to easily identify contents.

» **Get electric toothbrushes and shavers** to make hygiene tasks easier for your loved one to perform.

» **Substitute Velcro closures for buttons** on shirt cuffs, waistbands and other clothing that is hard to fasten. Some shoes also use Velcro!

» **Buy adaptive equipment** like covered cups, rocker knives, large-handled utensils and plate guards to make mealtime easier for your loved one.

» **Seek a referral to an occupational therapist** for individualized evaluation and recommendations tailored to your loved one's needs and concerns.

Visit Parkinson.org/library for a fact sheet on assistive devices.

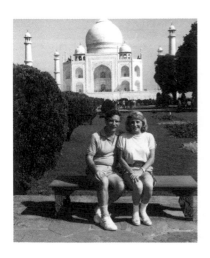

Jerry has had Parkinson's for more than 18 years, and I'm still struggling with finding balance. I'm still trying to be very idealistic, and it doesn't always work. You just have to go with the flow, and you have to say to yourself, 'We're going to get through this, and we're going to go onto the next step, and we're going to meet every challenge that we have to meet.'

– CAROLYN, CARES FOR HUSBAND, GERALD

Safety Considerations

As a caregiver, it can be difficult to recognize changes that occur slowly in the person with Parkinson's over time. If Parkinson's symptoms begin to significantly affect mobility, memory or thinking skills, it may be time to consider if it is still safe for your loved one to perform tasks that he or she once did easily as part of the daily routine.

While each person experiences Parkinson's differently, it is important to know that even familiar tasks can become difficult or unsafe for your loved one to continue. Making these changes can be difficult, so it is important for caregivers to acknowledge these losses and offer support as needed. Here are some examples:

DRIVING

Loss of flexibility in the neck and trunk, reduced reaction time and changes in ability to multi-task may affect your loved one's driving safety. Though it may be difficult to broach this topic, it is important to be realistic and seek medical advice and input if you notice changes. Occupational therapists are often involved in performing objective driving assessments and can offer recommendations based on their findings.

USE OF POWER TOOLS

Tremor combined with balance and coordination changes can impact safe use of power tools, even if the person with Parkinson's has used them for a long time. Slowed reaction time can also add to safety concerns. Consider all these factors when helping the person with Parkinson's determine if using power tools continues to be safe.

KITCHEN APPLIANCES

Cooking is often a multi-step process, and a person with Parkinson's may begin to have difficulty managing kitchen tasks safely. Balance changes can make opening refrigerator and oven doors difficult, and falls can occur when attempting to reach high shelves or carry objects from counter to table. You may need to change how the person with Parkinson's participates in the kitchen.

CLIMBING

Reductions in balance skills and protective reflexes increase falls risk in people with PD. Attempts to climb on ladders, step stools or other apparatus should be avoided, which may result in changes to tasks regularly performed in the house or yard.

Home Safety Tour Checklist

Use this checklist to ensure that your home is safe and easily accessible.

Throughout the House

☐ Floors are stable, non-skid surfaces without excessive patterns.

☐ There is good lighting throughout the home, with no dark or shadowy areas.

☐ Walking paths are wide, allowing easy access and use of a walker or wheelchair if needed.

☐ Electrical/phone/computer cords do not pose a tripping/falls risk when walking and moving about.

☐ Stairs are in good shape, have railings and can be blocked for safety if needed.

☐ Chairs are stable, have arm rests and adequate seat height to make standing up easier.

☐ Dining area can be easily accessed.

☐ A communication system is in place to allow you to hear the person with Parkinson's in another area of the house.

TO DO

☐ Remove throw rugs/scatter rugs.

☐ Remove clutter to decrease risk of tripping and falls.

☐ Store medication in a safe place.

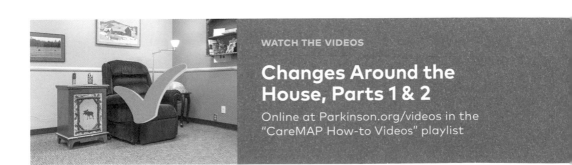

WATCH THE VIDEOS

Changes Around the House, Parts 1 & 2

Online at Parkinson.org/videos in the "CareMAP How-to Videos" playlist

Bedroom

- ☐ Environment is quiet and relaxing.
- ☐ Bed height allows feet to touch floor when seated at bedside.
- ☐ Half side rail or bed pole is in place to assist rolling and getting up.
- ☐ A nightlight is easily accessible and bright enough to fully light the path to the bathroom.
- ☐ A bedside commode/urinal is available for nighttime use if needed.
- ☐ A communication system or monitor is in place, so you can hear calls for help at night.

TO DO

- ☐ Place slippery fabric or a draw sheet on the middle third of the bed to make rolling easier.
- ☐ Remove the top sheet; instead, use a lightweight comforter.
- ☐ Avoid flannel sheets and nightwear.

Bathroom

- ☐ Grab bars are installed near the toilet, tub and shower: no location should require use of towel racks, faucets or soap dishes as grab bars.
- ☐ Toilet has an elevated seat and arm rests or grab bar within easy reach.
- ☐ Tub/shower has a sturdy bench with back support for bathing/shower safety.
- ☐ Seating is available if needed when performing tasks like brushing teeth, shaving, etc.
- ☐ A communication system or monitor is in place, if needed, so you can hear calls for help.

CHAPTER THREE: PRACTICAL POINTERS

Worksheets

Additional copies of any of these
worksheets may be downloaded from:
Parkinson.org/worksheets

Medical Appointment

Complete this form before each doctor's visit to help the person with Parkinson's fill out intake forms and make sure you get your top questions answered. Take notes to help you remember what is discussed at the appointment. Make copies of the blank form or download and print more so that you have one for each visit.

Top concerns:

1.

2.

3.

Bring a list of all medications that the person with Parkinson's is currently taking or write it below:

MEDICATION: ○ Need Refill

MEDICATION: ○ Need Refill

MEDICATION: ○ Need Refill

MEDICATION: ○ Need Refill

MEDICATION: ○ Need Refill

FILLED OUT BY: DATE:

Deep brain stimulation device? O No   O Yes

When was it implanted? _____

Illness, surgery / procedure, hospitalization, emergency room visits since last appointment? O No   O Yes

Describe: _____

_____

Current exercise routine: _____ _____

_____

Where does the person with Parkinson's live?
O Private home   O Apartment/condominium   O Assisted living
O Nursing home   O *Moved from last visit*

Does the person with Parkinson's live with someone?
O No   O Yes, with _____

Should a copy of dictation be sent to another doctor? O No   O Yes

Name: _____

Mailing address: _____

Use this space to take notes on what the doctor says:

_____

_____

_____

_____

_____

Medications and Schedule

Write in pencil so you can make changes more easily, or make copies of the blank form to update if there are medication changes.

MEDICATION NAME	PRESCRIBED FOR
EXAMPLE: Carb/levo 25/100	Parkinson's
EXAMPLE: Miralax	Constipation

FILLED OUT BY: DATE:

MEDICATION TIMES AND DOSE

AM PM	AM PM	AM PM	AM PM	AM PM	AM PM	COMMENTS / NOTES
	1.5 tab	1 tab	1.5 tab	1 tab	1.5 tab	
		X				1 scoop in 8 ounces of water

Parkinson's Symptoms Diary

Many symptoms of Parkinson's can be bothersome and interfere with day-to-day quality of life. Patient and family observations can help the medical team make a care plan. Fill out this worksheet and share it with providers to see if there is a pattern to when Parkinson's symptoms occur.

Morning

TIME	MEDICATION	MEAL	SLEEP
5:00 am			
5:30 am			
6:00 am			
6:30 am			
7:00 am			
7:30 am			
8:00 am			
8:30 am			
9:00 am			
9:30 am			
10:00 am			
10:30 am			
11:00 am			
11:30 am			

FILLED OUT BY: : DATE:

List the symptoms you want to track - e.g., tremor, dyskinesia, anxiety - in the top row.

When those symptoms occur, fill in the number that corresponds to the severity at that time.

Write medication names and doses next to the times at which the person with Parkinson's takes them.

Put an X (or list foods) in the "Meal" column at mealtimes.

Put an X in the "Sleep" column when the person with Parkinson's sleeps.

0 = NONE
1 = SLIGHT OR MILD
2 = MODERATE, BOTHERSOME
3 = SEVERE, VERY BOTHERSOME

SYMPTOMS   List 3

			NOTES
0 1 2 3	0 1 2 3	0 1 2 3	
0 1 2 3	0 1 2 3	0 1 2 3	
0 1 2 3	0 1 2 3	0 1 2 3	
0 1 2 3	0 1 2 3	0 1 2 3	
0 1 2 3	0 1 2 3	0 1 2 3	
0 1 2 3	0 1 2 3	0 1 2 3	
0 1 2 3	0 1 2 3	0 1 2 3	
0 1 2 3	0 1 2 3	0 1 2 3	
0 1 2 3	0 1 2 3	0 1 2 3	
0 1 2 3	0 1 2 3	0 1 2 3	
0 1 2 3	0 1 2 3	0 1 2 3	
0 1 2 3	0 1 2 3	0 1 2 3	
0 1 2 3	0 1 2 3	0 1 2 3	
0 1 2 3	0 1 2 3	0 1 2 3	

Afternoon & Evening

TIME	MEDICATION	MEAL	SLEEP
12:00 pm			
12:30 pm			
1:00 pm			
1:30 pm			
2:00 pm			
2:30 pm			
3:00 pm			
3:30 pm			
4:00 pm			
4:30 pm			
5:00 pm			
5:30 pm			
6:00 pm			
6:30 pm			
7:00 pm			
7:30 pm			
8:00 pm			

0 = NONE
1 = SLIGHT OR MILD
2 = MODERATE, BOTHERSOME
3 = SEVERE, VERY BOTHERSOME

SYMPTOMS   List 3

NOTES

0 1 2 3	0 1 2 3	0 1 2 3
0 1 2 3	0 1 2 3	0 1 2 3
0 1 2 3	0 1 2 3	0 1 2 3
0 1 2 3	0 1 2 3	0 1 2 3
0 1 2 3	0 1 2 3	0 1 2 3
0 1 2 3	0 1 2 3	0 1 2 3
0 1 2 3	0 1 2 3	0 1 2 3
0 1 2 3	0 1 2 3	0 1 2 3
0 1 2 3	0 1 2 3	0 1 2 3
0 1 2 3	0 1 2 3	0 1 2 3
0 1 2 3	0 1 2 3	0 1 2 3
0 1 2 3	0 1 2 3	0 1 2 3
0 1 2 3	0 1 2 3	0 1 2 3
0 1 2 3	0 1 2 3	0 1 2 3
0 1 2 3	0 1 2 3	0 1 2 3
0 1 2 3	0 1 2 3	0 1 2 3
0 1 2 3	0 1 2 3	0 1 2 3

Night

TIME	MEDICATION	MEAL	SLEEP
8:30 pm			
9:00 pm			
9:30 pm			
10:00 pm			
10:30 pm			
11:00 pm			
11:30 pm			
12:00 am			
12:30 am			
1:00 am			
1:30 am			
2:00 am			
2:30 am			
3:00 am			
3:30 am			
4:00 am			
4:30 am			

0 = NONE
1 = SLIGHT OR MILD
2 = MODERATE, BOTHERSOME
3 = SEVERE, VERY BOTHERSOME

SYMPTOMS List 3

			NOTES
0 1 2 3	0 1 2 3	0 1 2 3	
0 1 2 3	0 1 2 3	0 1 2 3	
0 1 2 3	0 1 2 3	0 1 2 3	
0 1 2 3	0 1 2 3	0 1 2 3	
0 1 2 3	0 1 2 3	0 1 2 3	
0 1 2 3	0 1 2 3	0 1 2 3	
0 1 2 3	0 1 2 3	0 1 2 3	
0 1 2 3	0 1 2 3	0 1 2 3	
0 1 2 3	0 1 2 3	0 1 2 3	
0 1 2 3	0 1 2 3	0 1 2 3	
0 1 2 3	0 1 2 3	0 1 2 3	
0 1 2 3	0 1 2 3	0 1 2 3	
0 1 2 3	0 1 2 3	0 1 2 3	
0 1 2 3	0 1 2 3	0 1 2 3	
0 1 2 3	0 1 2 3	0 1 2 3	
0 1 2 3	0 1 2 3	0 1 2 3	
0 1 2 3	0 1 2 3	0 1 2 3	

WORKSHEET

Notes:

CHAPTER FOUR

Caring from Afar

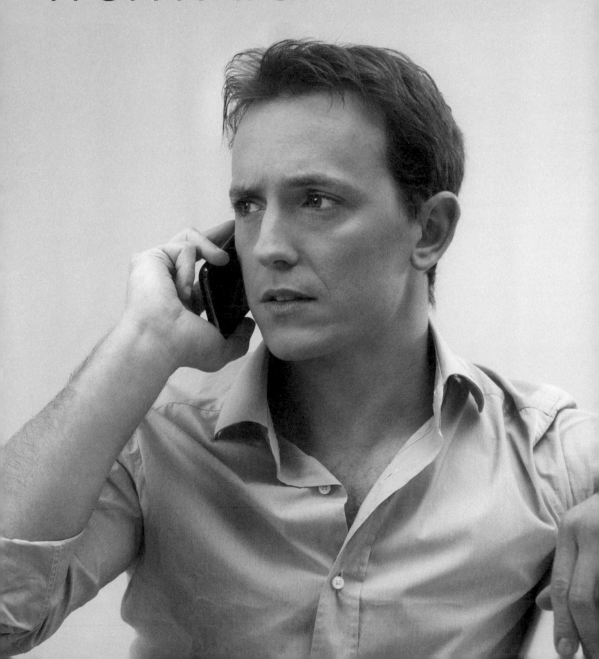

Caring from Afar

Parkinson's disease affects the whole family, whether you live in the same house as the person with Parkinson's or on another continent. In addition to tips for family caregivers who do not live in the same area as the person with Parkinson's, this section contains information for back-up, or secondary, caregivers: people who do live in the same place as the person with Parkinson's but are not the primary caregiver.

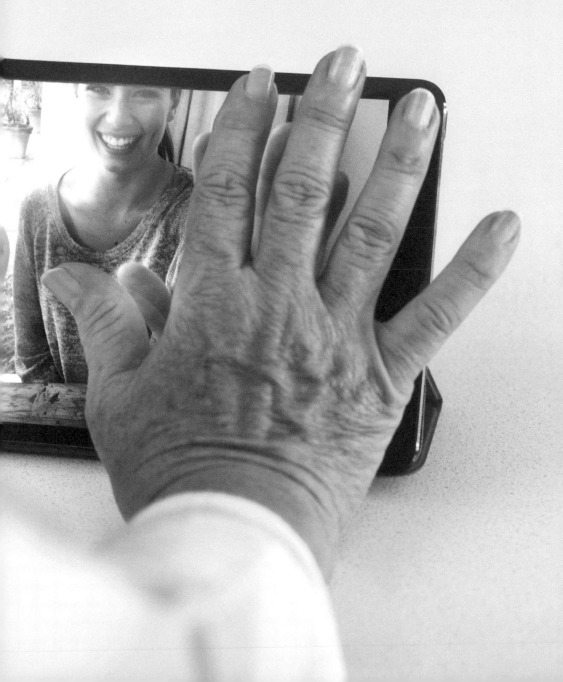

Secondary Caregiving

If you are a secondary caregiver, your role will never be as demanding as the one played by the primary caregiver – who may be a spouse/partner, sibling, adult child, other relative or friend of the person with Parkinson's. However, your role comes with its own unique rewards and challenges. Whether you are providing support from afar or act as back-up when the primary caregiver needs time off, there are many ways you can support both the person with PD and the primary caregiver. The following ideas will need to be adapted to your individual family and financial circumstances.

Call every week.
Set a designated day and time, and make the call faithfully. Inquire about both the person with PD and the caregiver. Make sure to include some topics not related to Parkinson's or caregiving to stay connected on multiple levels. Consider setting up Skype, FaceTime or another video call service so you can see each other on the call. Just be there to listen.

Find out if financial help is needed.
Many people will not ask for monetary help no matter how dire the situation. Inquire tactfully but clearly if expenses are a problem, and then offer a plan that can work for everyone. You could provide a regular monthly subsidy, cover a specific expense such as a month's supply of medications (especially important as long as the Medicare gap, or "donut hole," exists) or pay for a service that relieves the caregiver of one or more chores (e.g., housecleaning or yard services).

Send a care package once a month.
Try to tailor the surprise to the individual to make it more special. It might be a bouquet of favorite flowers, a magazine subscription for a personal interest or a gift card to buy something just for them. Be creative. Never underestimate how much a personally written thank-you note can mean to a caregiver whose work goes mostly unrecognized.

Visit the person with Parkinson's.
Budget time and funds for regular visits. Find your own way from the airport, and book a hotel room if quarters are cramped. Your trip should not add to the responsibilities and strain of the primary caregiver. Make the goal of your visit to provide a listening ear and a helping hand. Spending time with the caregiver and the person with Parkinson's will give you a firsthand look at specific challenges and issues and help you think about how to be involved.

Try to schedule at least one of your visits when the person with Parkinson's has an appointment with the neurologist. This will allow you to better understand your loved one's medical status, see how the doctor, patient and caregiver interact and add your own valuable observations. During your visit, remember to ask about the health of the caregiver. Are regular check-ups and screenings being overlooked because of caregiving responsibilities? Consider coordinating a visit so the caregiver can schedule doctor, dentist and optometrist visits while you stay with the person with Parkinson's.

Provide respite for the primary caregiver.
If you cannot fill in personally, locate other options and offer to cover the costs if possible. There may be free or low-cost services available that the primary caregiver just hasn't had the energy to locate. Many people who care for someone with Parkinson's say that their role started much earlier in the course of the disease than anyone else realized. If your loved one is able to travel, invite him or her for a visit. This allows the person with Parkinson's to get all your attention and enjoy a change of scenery while the primary caregiver enjoys a welcome break in familiar surroundings.

Support the healthcare team's and primary caregiver's decisions.
Express vocal support to your loved one for the healthcare team's care and safety recommendations, such as using a walker, not driving, accepting additional help with personal care or wearing a medical identification bracelet. Similarly, if and when the time comes, affirm the difficult decision to place your loved one in a care facility. Be respectful of the fact that you are not the person providing day-to-day care. You may not fully recognize how caregiving responsibilities have grown. It is a mistake to let worries about cash flow, sibling rivalry or dwindling inheritances get in the way of doing what is best for the people whose lives are most affected.

What Not to Do

It might feel like you need permission to help, like the primary caregiver cannot or will not delegate responsibilities. This can be frustrating and emotional. Use the strategies on the previous pages to support from afar, and avoid these common mistakes:

Not understanding the severity of day-to-day symptoms.
Many caregivers will say that the person with Parkinson's is at his or her best when at a doctor's appointment or having visitors. What you see when you visit may be quite different from the daily reality. Research found that people who care for someone with Parkinson's provided an average of 14 hours of care daily and had greater levels of physical and emotional strain than people caring for someone with Alzheimer's disease.

Offering too much unsolicited advice.
Friends and relatives who do not provide daily care often have a valuable ability to "see the forest instead of the trees." However, this objective wisdom must be expressed with great care and without criticism for family members who live close by and carry the greater responsibility of caregiving.

Not honoring the historical relationship of the caregiver and the person with Parkinson's.
In most cases, the caregiver and the person with Parkinson's will have had a long and intimate relationship with one another. One caregiving wife said to her daughter, "My relationship with your father may be dysfunctional, but it's OUR dysfunctional relationship." Trying to make fundamental changes in a relationship of many years can result in frustration and hurt feelings for everyone involved.

COMMUNICATION TIPS

» When talking with the caregiver or the person with Parkinson's, **always listen to what is being said** instead of thinking about what you are going to say next.

» **Be especially careful when sending email or text messages.** Without the benefit of eye contact and body language, messages can be misunderstood and feelings can be hurt.

» **Do not expect any of your loved one's healthcare team to speak with you** unless the person with Parkinson's has signed a release giving his or her permission.

» **Remember to ask the primary caregiver what he or she would find helpful.** It may be that paying the bills and balancing the checkbook is more important than a cleaning service.

» **Not all problems can be solved.** Sometimes the caregiver needs a patient, understanding ear rather than a quick solution.

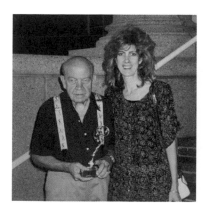

There's guilt when you are away from your loved one. The primary caregiver is at home when you're not. You love the person as much as they do, but for whatever reason you can't be there every day. There's sadness that goes along with that because you want to be there.

– KAREN, CARED FOR FATHER, JOSEPH

Primary Caregiving from Afar

Many primary long-distance caregivers enter into this relationship because their loved ones do not want to leave their home or environment. This is understandable. But Parkinson's is a progressive, degenerative illness. At some point, your loved one may need in-home care or relocation to an assisted living or skilled nursing facility.

Unless you are able to make frequent visits, have friends or other relatives who can visit often and report back to you or have the finances to hire a geriatric care manager, you may need to move the person with Parkinson's closer to you to assure that he or she receives consistent and adequate care. Since travel can become more difficult as the disease progresses, a move should be discussed sooner rather than later.

If the person lives alone, consider daily well-being calls or checks by a neighbor. The call should be set for a specific time every day when the person is most likely to be home. If there is a neighbor that is willing to do so, you can alternate calls and visits. You might also want to consider an emergency alert system, especially since falls are so prevalent in advancing Parkinson's.

Educate Yourself
Learn all about Parkinson's, including motor and non-motor symptoms, the drugs used to treat the disease and other available forms of treatment. You must be well-versed in the needs and functional status of the person with Parkinson's. You may wish to hire a geriatric care manager to conduct a functional assessment every six months. These assessments determine how well the individual is able to perform activities of daily living such as bathing and dressing and instrumental activities of daily living such as taking medications properly and preparing meals.

Learn about your loved one's general health and all medications taken including dosages, regimes and possible side effects. Keep a list of your loved one's doctors, specialists, pharmacist, care providers and neighbors along with contact information. Keep all financial and legal documents easily accessible and make sure bills are paid in a timely manner. Parkinson's disease and some of the medications used to treat it can result in compulsive behaviors. Try to find a discrete way to monitor any gambling activities as well as excessive spending or eating.

Keep in Touch

If for whatever reason you cannot move your loved one closer to you, communicate regularly with the person with Parkinson's and his or her local care providers, whether that means an in-home aide or the staff at a care facility. If your loved one's needs change, you need to know what that will mean for him or her – more skilled in-home care, visits with a different medical specialist, additional prescriptions, new diet regimens – as well as what it will mean for you – more visits, higher costs for care, etc. You can help assess changing needs during each visit.

Work with a Geriatric Care Manager

A geriatric care manager can provide a number of useful services for a fee. These services include regular wellbeing checks, ongoing communication with family members and arranging financial, legal and medical services, in-home care providers and transportation. Fees vary depending on what services are needed. You should personally interview the prospective care manager, ideally during one of your visits, before engaging his or her services.

The Aging Life Care Association offers a Certified Geriatric Care Manager designation to those who have been certified by one of three certifying bodies and who have completed the Association's necessary education and work experience requirements. Make sure to obtain proof of certification before hiring someone.

Be Kind to Yourself

Caregiving from a distance can be emotionally taxing, so make sure you have a support system in place.

Visit the "Caring for You" section at **Parkinson.org/caregivers** *to find tips and tools for self-care.*

COMMUNICATION TIPS

» Make sure the person with Parkinson's has **signed the necessary forms** with all of the medical personnel providing care.

» **Include other topics in your conversation** with your loved one so that every call is not always just about Parkinson's.

» **Remember to show appreciation often** to everyone involved in the care of the person with Parkinson's – neighbors, volunteers, friends and paid personnel.

» **If moving your loved one closer is an eventual goal, start talking about this early and gently.** It is always preferable to reach a mutual agreement rather than imposing your will.

» **Try to offer care solutions that provide as much autonomy as possible.** Remember that a mentally competent adult has the right to make choices for himself or herself as long as those choices do not put others at risk. This ability to make choices comes with responsibility for the consequences of those choices.

CHAPTER FIVE

Getting Outside Help

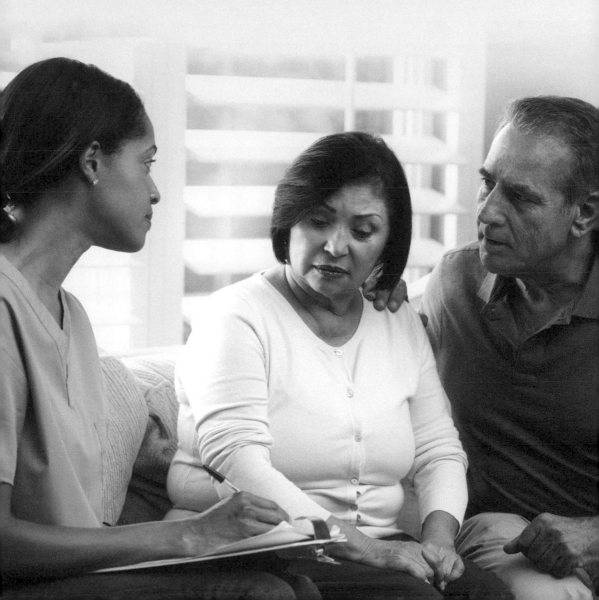

Getting Outside Help

In too many instances, long-term caregiving takes place without necessary knowledge or support. Don't let this happen to you! Begin adding outside resources to your caregiving early on. This makes adding other care sources easier as the disease progresses. This section will help you decide when it's time to get help, where to find additional help, how to utilize paid caregivers and when to consider moving the person with Parkinson's out of the home.

IN THIS CHAPTER

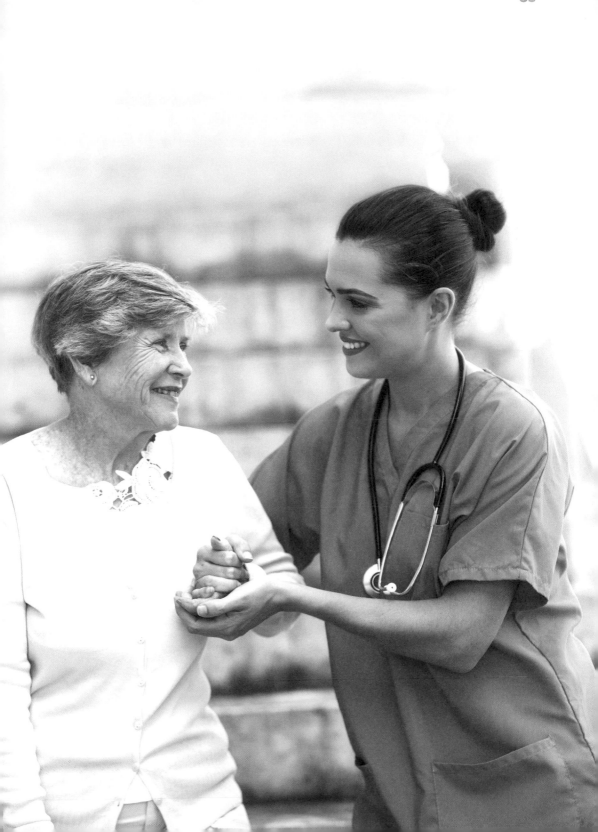

When Is It Time to Get Help?

It has been said that Parkinson's is a family disease – that is, when someone is diagnosed, everyone in the family is affected. Hopefully from the beginning there has been a variety of people involved in meeting the needs of the person with Parkinson's – needs for socialization, emotional support, education, love and more. No one person is ever able to meet all of an individual's needs, and as Parkinson's progresses this becomes more and more true.

As your loved one's care needs change, you must continually reevaluate your need for help. At first you might just need someone to help pick up groceries every now and then. As the disease advances, your needs might evolve to include a day care service or a home health aide for a few hours at a time. Eventually, full-time home care or a skilled nursing facility might be necessary.

One of the first ways to relieve some of the stress of caring for someone with Parkinson's is to add others into the caregiving mix. Take advantage of your network of friends and family. Most people get a good feeling when they are able to help someone. When someone asks how they can help, have a list of ideas to suggest. Even occasional help eases the task of caregiving. See the worksheet "Adding Friends, Family and Volunteers to Your Caregiving" on page 106 for ideas on how this might be done.

The best time to investigate in-home care options as well as adult day programs and other services is BEFORE those options are needed. This will make your life easier if these transitions become necessary in the future.

DEVELOP AN EMERGENCY PLAN

If you are the primary caregiver, it is important that you have an emergency plan for your loved one's care should you become sick or temporarily disabled. Knowledge of outside resources is vital to making your plan. Knowing what will happen if something happens to you also provides security for the person with Parkinson's.

Be Realistic

Many people make promises to always care for their loved one themselves, at home. These promises are often asked for and made even before the person develops any health concerns. If you are asked to make this promise, affirm your commitment and support for the person's desire to remain at home as long as it is safe and practical to do so.

If you have already made this promise, you may not have understood all the responsibilities that caregiving entails. For example, in late-stage Parkinson's, many people cannot help with their own movements or activities of daily living, and falls can become more serious and frequent. This means regular heavy lifting.

You might feel like a traitor if you have to break your promise because you don't have the physical strength or stamina – or the technical skills – to provide the kind of care the person with Parkinson's needs. It is best to discuss, in advance of need, the situations that may arise that will not allow you to keep your promise. Also talk about various care alternatives that may become necessary, and encourage the person with Parkinson's to tell you which scenarios are most acceptable.

Sometimes people with Parkinson's refuse to let anyone besides the primary caregiver provide help. Or, if outside help is brought in, the person with Parkinson's insists that the primary caregiver remain at home. This is unrealistic and unsafe for both you and your loved one. Have a straight-forward conversation with the person with Parkinson's about what will happen to him or her if something happens to you. It may seem easier in the short run to put up with these demands rather than go through bouts of arguments and poor behavior. However, with resolve and continued exposure to outside care, the person with Parkinson's will eventually come around.

Ultimately, when it becomes too difficult to balance your own life with your caregiving responsibilities, when the safety of the care recipient is in question or when the physical burden is more than you are capable of, it is time to get outside help.

Where to Find Help

Getting outside help does not necessarily mean hiring services through a home care agency or private in-home caregiver.

Who Can Help

THE NATIONAL FAMILY CAREGIVER SUPPORT PROGRAM (NFCSP)

Established in 2000, this program provides grants to states and territories, based on their share of the population aged 70 and over, to fund a range of supports that assist family and informal caregivers to care for their loved ones at home for as long as possible. The care recipient must be 60 years of age or older.

Services include:
- Information to caregivers about available services
- Assistance to caregivers in gaining access to the services
- Individual counseling, organization of support groups and caregiver training
- Respite care
- Supplemental services, on a limited basis

To access this program as well as other state-based programs, contact your local Area Agency on Aging (AAA). Your local AAA can also provide information on adult day care, case management, home modification, home health services and much more. They will let you know whether services are free or available on a sliding fee scale. To find your local AAA:

Eldercare Locator Service
www.eldercare.gov
1-800-677-1116

VETERANS ADMINISTRATION CAREGIVER SERVICES
1-855-260-3274 (8 AM to 8 PM Eastern Time, Monday – Friday)

Contact the VA to learn what assistance might be available for veterans and their spouses or widow(er)s. The call center is staffed by licensed social workers who can explain available services, give you contact information for accessing those services and provide emotional support. Most of the services are income- or asset-based, and it may take from six months to a year for approval. Payment is retroactive to date of filing.

VOLUNTEERS

The National Volunteer Caregiving Network (formerly Faith in Action) exists to share knowledge, experiences and ideas that help strengthen and support hundreds of local volunteer caregiving programs throughout the U.S. and to foster the establishment of new interfaith volunteer caregiving programs. Their website (www.nvcnetwork.org) allows you to search by state to see what volunteer caregiving programs are available near you. If you do not have internet access, call their national office for help finding the nearest program: 512-582-2197. Individual programs will explain what services are offered and the limitations of those services.

You should also check if your town has a volunteer agency; the agency will do background checks and training before assigning volunteers. Many college and even high school students participate in community service organizations. Faith-based youth groups, young professionals and retired people also like to volunteer in the community. Depending on their level of comfort and your own, these volunteers might be able to help with a variety of tasks, from grocery shopping to light housekeeping to basic caregiving.

IN-HOME CARE PROVIDERS

Home healthcare agencies may be affiliated with hospitals and focus on the medical aspects of care. Services from these agencies are generally limited by insurance or Medicare to a certain number of visits.

Home care agencies provide non-medical services including personal care, housekeeping, companionship and supervision. Their services may be short or long-term. Unless you have a long-term care insurance policy that covers in-home care or certain VA benefits, the cost of these services will be out-of-pocket to you.

LOCAL PARKINSON'S FOUNDATION CHAPTER

Some Parkinson's Foundation Chapters offer respite grants. All will be able to refer you to service providers in your area. Visit **Parkinson.org/search** or call our Helpline at 1-800-4PD-INFO (473-4636) to see if we have a Chapter near you.

Action Plan for Hiring In-Home Caregivers

First and foremost, you want someone who is able to perform all the caregiving tasks you need accomplished. You also want someone who can form a comfortable working relationship with both you and the person with Parkinson's. Take your time and select carefully.

» **Define your loved one's and your caregiving needs.** Do you need help with bathing and respite care a couple times a week? Do you need someone available eight hours every night to help the person with Parkinson's to the bathroom and supervise him or her so you can get uninterrupted sleep?

» **Develop a job description.** Include a list of household tasks, personal care tasks and leisure activities that the home care worker will be expected to do. A well-developed job description will help you or an agency assure that the right worker is hired. It can also be used as a basis to evaluate the worker and, if necessary, terminate employment.

» **Find out about legal, financial and tax issues.** Check with your insurance agent to determine whether your homeowner's policy covers property damage, theft and personal injury that involves an employee or other person working in the home. Does your automobile insurance cover a home care worker driving the family car, and if so, are there any exceptions? Read "Deciding to Hire Through an Agency or Privately" on page 92 for more in-depth information on legal and tax issues.

» **Screen and interview applicants.** If you are hiring privately, you will first want to interview candidates by phone, then set up in-person interviews with the most promising ones. Have the job description ready to hand them and a formal list of questions. Remember to include any individual preferences or behaviors that might preclude certain work, such as "this is a smoking household," "my loved one will not accept personal care from a man/woman," "the person with Parkinson's often swears," etc. If you are hiring from an agency, you may only be presented with one candidate at a time. Presumably the agency has used the information you provided in their care planning interview to pick the best match for your needs. If you truly do not think this person will fit into your household, tell the agency, and ask them to send someone else.

» **Check references and backgrounds.** Whether hiring an agency to provide your home care worker or hiring privately, it is vital that you ask for at least two references. Check them! The agency should have done a criminal background check on their employees, but you will need to do one if you hire privately.

» **Sign a contract or care provider agreement.** If you are using an agency, they will supply a contract that shows what services have been contracted, what rate will be charged, any charges for additional services and billing and payment information. If you hire privately, you should have a written agreement that specifically outlines the terms of employment including salary, days and hours of service, any benefits (e.g., paid holidays, provision of meals, etc.), work rules and notice required for either party to terminate the agreement. Both parties to any contract or agreement should be given a copy for their records.

» **If you decide to hire someone privately, you can place an ad in your local paper or search online.** There are many websites that specialize in providing care services, from companion care to personal care to around-the-clock care. You might also look for a placement agency. These companies charge a one-time finder's fee for placing a caregiver in a home. The caregivers are often from other countries and may have limited English proficiency. Whichever option you choose, you should make sure the person is legally able to work in the U.S.

The worksheets "Questions to Ask a Potential Paid Agency and Individual Caregiver" on pages 110 and 112 can help you select either an agency or individual.

Deciding to Hire Through an Agency or Privately

There are pros and cons for deciding to use an agency or hire in-home caregiving help privately. Here are the ABCs you need to consider.

ADMINISTRATION

Hiring privately involves running ads, screening applicants, doing background checks, verifying that the person is eligible to work in the U.S., doing payroll including filing forms and paying taxes at regular intervals during the year, supervising, evaluating and, if necessary, firing the worker.

BACKUP

If the worker becomes ill or has a family emergency, who will provide service? Agencies usually can provide another worker relatively quickly; this may not be true for someone you hire privately.

BONDING

This is an insurance policy that protects both the employee and the employer against financial loss. Agencies usually bond their employees. Should you bond your privately hired worker? Check with your insurance agent to find out what is involved.

COST

In most cases, hiring privately will cost less than hiring through an agency.

CONSISTENCY

An agency may not be able to provide the same person every time. You may end up having to train several workers.

DID YOU KNOW? ....

According to research from the *Parkinson's Outcomes Project*, the largest clinical study of Parkinson's ever conducted, women with Parkinson's have less informal caregiving support from spouses and other family members and are twice as likely as men to have a paid caregiver.

INDEPENDENT CONTRACTOR STATUS

Independent contractors are responsible for reporting their income and paying their own Social Security and Medicare taxes. Some caregivers and workers want to claim this status to avoid paperwork and/or paying taxes. This is often the case if you hire through a placement agency that uses foreign workers. The Internal Revenue Service (IRS) has strict requirements for individuals operating as independent contractors. The IRS rule is, "Anyone who performs services is an employee if you (the employer) can control what will be done and how it will be done – what matters is that you have the legal right to control the method and result of the services."

Hiring someone as an independent contractor might affect your ability to deduct in-home care expenses as part of your medical expense deductions and might also affect payment from a long-term care insurance policy that covers in-home care. You should check with your tax preparer and your long-term insurance agent before hiring someone with independent contractor status.

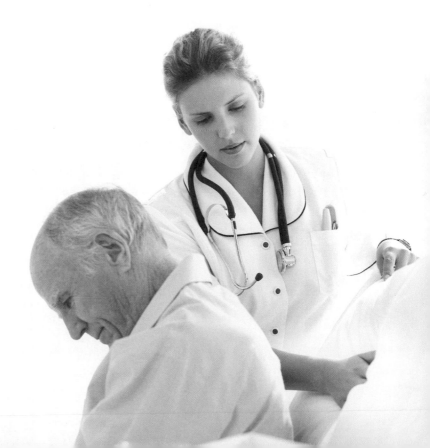

Preparing Paid Caregivers

Leaving the care of your loved one in someone else's hands is not easy. But if you hire the right person and familiarize them with your loved one's particular needs, it can be an invaluable help.

It is important for the people or agency you hire to understand Parkinson's, so they can understand and better relate to your loved one. Even seasoned professionals might not know about Parkinson's disease. You can provide the agency and/or worker with the free book *What You and Your Family Should Know*. The worksheet "Orienting a New Home Care Worker" on page 108 will give you more information to help make sure that you and the worker get off to a good start.

Getting to Know the Person with Parkinson's
Once they know about the disease, paid caregivers need to get to know the person. To provide the best possible care for the person with Parkinson's, it is helpful for home care workers to understand the person's history, personality and preferences as well as the family situation. Explain or provide a written document with insights on your loved one's childhood, occupation, family stories, favorite hobbies, likes, dislikes and daily routines. Include information on relatives or friends who are involved in caring for the person with Parkinson's.

Make a Care Plan
With this understanding in place, you, the person with Parkinson's and the home care worker should collaborate to develop a care plan and checklist. It is important to identify and discuss the care and support needs of the person with Parkinson's. These needs, and the steps that will be taken to address them, should be written down in a manner that is easily understood by all who are providing daily care and assistance. This document (referred to as a care plan) can help ensure that all necessary steps are taken to provide the best possible care on an ongoing basis.

Keep in Touch
If you are not living in the home with the care recipient, communication is key to better care. Make sure to check in regularly with the home care workers, particularly as your loved one's needs change over time. The care plan will need to be updated to reflect the progression of Parkinson's disease, so this is a good time to evaluate the caregiver relationship. Voice any concerns about the quality of care being provided. Stay calm and respectful during the conversation, but follow up to make sure that problems are addressed.

COMMUNICATION TIPS

» **Short sentences** that use everyday vocabulary lead to better understanding.

» **When correcting a worker, focus the discussion on the work.** Emphasize the actions and the behavior, not the person or the personality.

» **Avoid "you" statements and the words "always" and "never."** Telling someone "you always" or "you never" is a set-up for an argument.

» **Provide frequent, meaningful and specific praise.** Include details of what was done and why you appreciated it.

» **Seek regular feedback from the care worker.** Ask how the job is going, what concerns he or she may have, suggestions for improving care and how you can be helpful. Remember to listen to the answers before formulating your response. If you hear something upsetting, ask for time to think about it before responding, but make sure you do respond.

Know the Roles

Paid caregivers are hired to keep the person with Parkinson's safe and look after his or her well-being. Caregiver and care recipient might form a bond over time, but it is important that paid caregivers maintain professional boundaries. They should not become involved in familial or financial conversations and decision-making. While your role as a family caregiver is emotional and complex, remember that no matter how nice the home care worker is or how much she or he likes you or the person with Parkinson's, it is a job.

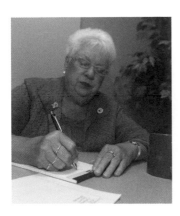

I needed to provide some training with every single aide that came in that was going to stay all night. I had to talk to them about Rogers' personality, show them where things were and how he moves and what would help them move him, just a lot of logistics and little things about him.

– LENNORE, CARED FOR HUSBAND, ROGER

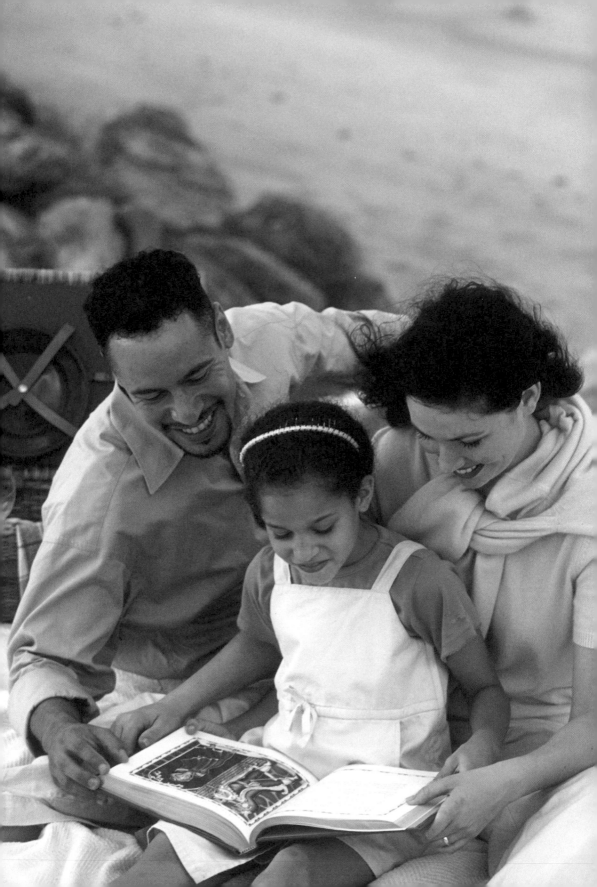

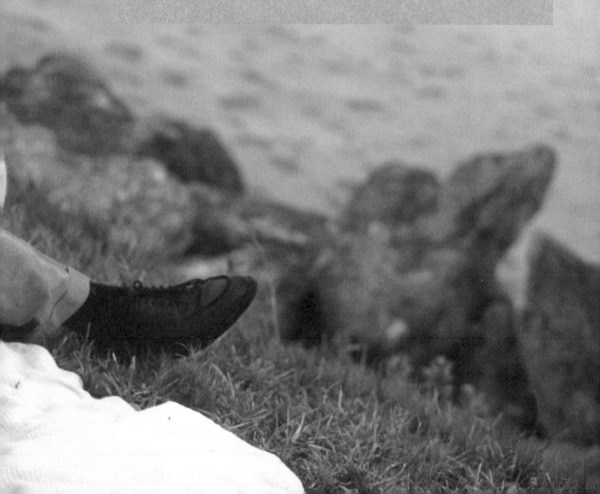

Make a date with friends or family.

Spending time with people you love provides stimulation and support for you and the person with Parkinson's.

Respite Care

What is respite care?

"Respite" means a short period of relief. "Respite care" refers to short-term, temporary care provided to your loved one so you can take a break from the daily routine of caregiving.

Caregiving is a tough job with long hours. To maintain your physical and emotional health and provide the best care for the person with Parkinson's, respite is essential and is often referred to as "a gift of time." Respite care enables families to take time off, for a few hours or even multiple days.

Who provides respite services, and what kinds of services are provided?

INFORMAL, PERSONAL ARRANGEMENTS

Prepare and train a couple friends or family members to fill in for you. You should have more than one option in case someone is not available.

FORMAL SERVICES

The two primary categories of respite include in-home services and out-of-home services. Depending on the provider, the needs of the family and available funds, the following are typical services provided in each category:

IN-HOME RESPITE

With home-based services, a trained, licensed, insured and bonded employee of a private or state agency comes to the home. Services are generally available 24 hours a day, 365 days a year. In-home care refers to personal care with activities of daily living, such as bathing, grooming and dressing. In-home care providers are also called companions, personal aides or personal caregivers. They work either for themselves privately or for an agency that takes responsibility for setting fees, making caregiving assignments, insuring and bonding the caregivers and training them. In-home caregivers can be employed to assist with a particular task – for example, bathing assistance – or by blocks of time – four hours, eight hours or even live-in.

For the most part, personal care is a private expense. Medicare or health insurance does not cover it. However, it may be covered by your long-term care insurance policy. Many states, through their local Area Agencies on Aging, offer a capped number of hours of companion services to older adults.

OUT-OF-HOME RESPITE

Family Care Homes: In this case, respite is provided in someone's home. Homes and the care providers should be licensed under state regulations to provide housing, meals and personal care services to the elderly and others.

Adult Day Programs: These programs (also referred to as adult day care) are community-based, day-long social and recreational programs provided in a safe, secure group setting. Such programs may be held in churches and synagogues, community centers, park districts, healthcare institutions or other facilities. Most programs offer some health-related services, such as medication reminders. Adult day programs may also include the following:

- Transportation
- Meals and snacks
- Assistance with, or supervision of, eating, walking and toileting
- Exercise
- Socialization and peer support
- Social work services
- On-site or on-call nurse

In addition to the benefits to participants, adult day programs afford family caregivers a respite from the demands of full-time caregiving for someone who needs constant supervision. Services and fees for adult day vary from program to program and state to state.

Residential Facilities: As well as serving as permanent residences, many long-term residential facilities have a specified number of rooms set aside for short-term respite.

My friends and family remind me that if I don't take care of myself, I will not be able to care for Irving. He attends an adult day center once a week, and I attend care partner support group twice a month. These things are truly a lifesaver.

– MARIE, CARES FOR IRVING

How do caregivers benefit from respite services?

Beyond direct relief, the benefits of respite care can also include the following:

- **Relaxation:** Families can relax, gain peace of mind and renew their humor and energy.

- **Enjoyment:** Families can enjoy favorite pastimes and pursue new activities.

- **Stability:** Respite can improve the family's ability to cope with daily responsibilities and maintain stability during crisis.

- **Preservation:** Respite helps preserve the family unit and lessens the pressures that might lead to institutionalization, divorce, neglect and abuse.

- **Involvement:** Families can become involved in community activities and be less isolated.

- **Time off:** Families can take a needed vacation, spend time together or spend time alone.

- **Enrichment:** Respite makes it possible for family members to establish individual identities and enrich their own growth and development.

What do you need to know when seeking respite services in your community?
Here are some questions you may want to ask yourself when considering respite services:

- What kind of services do I need (long- or short-term or both), and why?
- Do I prefer services in my home or an outside setting?
- Does the agency provide the type of services I need?
- What is the cost of services? How is payment arranged?
- What is the training and level of experience of the care providers? Will they need additional training to meet the specific needs of my loved one?
- How, and by whom, are the care providers supervised?
- Does the program maintain current information about clients' medical and other needs? Is there a written care plan?
- What procedures does the program have for emergencies?
- Can family members meet and interview the people who care for the person with Parkinson's?
- How far ahead of time do I need to call to arrange for services?
- Are families limited to a certain number of hours of service?
- Does the program provide transportation?

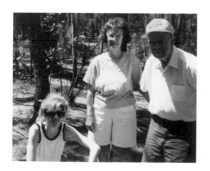

So many caregivers are so wrapped up in what they're doing for the person that they love, that they totally neglect themselves - and in doing so they are not the best caregiver they can be.

– KAREN, CARED FOR FATHER, JOSEPH

Rehabilitation and Parkinson's Disease

Skilled rehabilitation therapies – including physical therapy, occupational therapy and speech therapy – can help a person with Parkinson's maintain or re-stabilize functioning and offer helpful safety instructions for the caregiver.

These therapies are provided in multiple settings: day treatment centers, your home, in-patient units of rehabilitation institutions and out-patient centers. Skilled therapy is an order prescribed by a physician. It is covered by Medicare and other health insurance companies, so long as the person is not already receiving insurance-covered therapies in more than one setting at the same time.

IN-PATIENT REHABILITATION

Large, dedicated rehabilitation institutions offer in-patient rehab stays as well as all other levels of rehab treatment. To qualify for an in-patient rehab unit, the person with Parkinson's must meet specific criteria related to the ability to participate in and benefit from multiple daily, intensive therapy sessions.

OUT-PATIENT THERAPY

Out-patient therapy is provided in a community clinic setting, so your loved one must be able to leave the home for therapy. The person with Parkinson's receives a one-hour session of physical, occupational or speech therapy.

DAY REHABILITATION PROGRAMS

In addition to in-patient and out-patient rehabilitation, some rehabilitation institutions offer day rehabilitation: a concentrated, rather intense, community-based, day-long treatment program that encompasses all of the skilled rehabilitation therapies: physical, occupational and speech. To qualify, the person with Parkinson's must be able to undertake three hours of therapies in a day.

IN-HOME THERAPY

In-home therapy refers to physician-ordered, skilled rehabilitation therapy – physical, occupational or speech – for patients who are home-bound and unable to travel to an out-patient therapy setting. A registered nurse opens and oversees the home rehabilitation care. During the time that a case is open for home rehab, your loved one is also eligible to receive a bath aide. However, the bath service ends when the course of rehabilitation ends.

CHAPTER FIVE: GETTING OUTSIDE HELP

Worksheets

Additional copies of any of these
worksheets may be downloaded from:
Parkinson.org/worksheets

Daily Routine

Complete this worksheet so that anyone who fills in for you as caregiver will know how to care for the person with Parkinson's.

Usually arises at: _____

Usually goes to bed at: _____

It is very important that Parkinson's medications are given on time every time, according to schedule.
See the Medications Worksheet for more information.

Are there allergies to any foods or substances?

_____

_____

Are there dietary restrictions or food/beverage consistencies needed? Favorite foods/dislikes?

_____

_____

Are any special adaptations used for eating, dressing or personal cares?

_____

_____

Hobbies and interests:

_____

_____

FILLED OUT BY: DATE:

What is the typical daily routine? Include mealtime, activities, rest periods, exercise, personal cares and other activities.

_____

_____

_____

_____

_____

_____

_____

Additional information:

_____

_____

_____

_____

_____

_____

_____

_____

_____

_____

Adding Family, Friends and Volunteers to Your Caregiving

Take advantage of your network and the kindness of others, but be mindful of potential schedule conflicts and time constraints. Consider having several options or a back-up plan in case your regular assistance is unable to help. Be honest, open and specific regarding what is needed when you ask for and accept help from those who are close to you. Even the healthiest families can be stressed by long-term care. It can help to keep everyone up-to-date on your loved one's needs and condition.

PERSON TO ASK	ACTIVITY
EXAMPLE: Jack's brother Tom	Take Jack to Lunch
EXAMPLE: Neighbor Jim	Take garbage out
EXAMPLE: Volunteer Sally Smith	Respite

FILLED OUT BY: DATE:

Different people will have different skills and preferences for how they help out. Help may not always involve direct caregiving. Someone who is willing to cut the grass every week frees up your time or money to use in another way.

Enlisting the help of volunteers will allow you to diversify your support system but will also require flexibility and coordination on your part. The below chart can help you decide who you can ask, what job that person can do, and what the time commitment would be.

CONTACT (PHONE OR EMAIL)	TIME COMMITMENT
tom@email.com	Once a week, 90 minutes
555-1212	Once a week, 10 minutes
sally@email.com	Once a week, 2 hours

Orienting a New Home Care Worker

If you have never had paid staff in your home, you might not know how to orient and train someone you hire. In *Home Health Aides, How to Manage the People Who Help You*, Alfred DeGraff identifies five mistakes that can create problems between you and your worker:

- **Not providing clear instructions**

- **Expecting the worker to provide duties that were not agreed upon or adding extra tasks at the last minute**

- **Not recognizing work well done**

- **Comparing them unfavorably to other workers**

- **Being either too critical or too passive when providing feedback**

When training a worker to do a task, use this five-step process:

1) Tell the worker how to do the task.

2) Show the worker how to do the task.

3) Have the worker perform the task while you observe.

4) Praise progress.

5) Provide an opportunity to ask questions, and make sure the worker understands your answers.

The checklist at right can be used to help you provide a good orientation. Review all the information listed with the new worker. Also remember to show the worker the layout of the home, where the things he or she will need to do the job are kept and how to operate appliances or medical devices.

FILLED OUT BY: : DATE:

ORIENTATION TASK

☐ Demonstrate how tasks should be done

☐ Information about the household routines

☐ Review emergency procedures and whom to contact

☐ Information about the care recipient's preferences
(e.g., prefers formal address "Mr. Smith" – not "honey")

☐ Clear instructions about what is out of bounds
(e.g., having visitors, changing the thermostat, smoking)

☐ A clear procedure for keeping track of cash dispensed and spent
if the worker is responsible for shopping or other activities that
require cash

☐ How to prevent/respond to potential problems such as wandering

☐ Information about what the person with Parkinson's enjoys doing
and what he or she is able to do independently

☐ Caregiving tips peculiar to your loved one – this allows the worker to
create a pleasant atmosphere and avoid doing anything disturbing

Notes:

Questions to Ask a Potential Paid Individual Caregiver

Hiring someone to take care of your loved one is a decision that must be made with careful consideration. There are many questions you can ask to make sure the individual can meet your needs, as well as questions to make sure the person is competent and has the proper training, licensing and insurance.

POTENTIAL CAREGIVER NAME:

What is your education and training?

_____

_____

IF INDIVIDUAL IS A SKILLED PROVIDER (RN, PT, OT, SLP, SW):
Do you provide both medical and non-medical services?

O No O Yes _____

What hours are you available?

_____

_____

Are you licensed/certified by any government agency to provide home care?

O No O Yes _____

Do you carry liability insurance?

O No O Yes _____

Will you perform an in-home assessment prior to starting service?

O No O Yes _____

Will you create a care plan?

O No O Yes _____

Is there a process for updating the services provided if our needs change?

O No O Yes _____

Can you provide in writing the care services provided and clearly describe all rates and fees?

O No O Yes _____

What are your fees?

_____

_____

What is the billing schedule for services?

_____

_____

What happens if you become ill or are otherwise unavailable? What are the alternate arrangements?

_____

_____

How do you document that your services were completed?

_____

_____

How quickly can you initiate service?

_____

_____

Can you provide a list of references?

O No O Yes _____

_____

Questions to Ask a Potential Paid Agency Caregiver

Hiring someone to take care of your loved one is a decision that must be made with careful consideration. There are many questions you can ask to make sure the agency can meet your needs, as well as questions to make sure the agency and its employees are competent and have the proper training, licensing and insurance.

POTENTIAL CAREGIVER/AGENCY NAME:

Questions About Services Provided

Does your agency provide both medical services (such as skilled nursing, rehab therapies, etc.) and non-medical services (such as bathing, incontinence care and mobility assistance)?

○ No ○ Yes _____

Will you perform an in-home assessment prior to starting service?

○ No ○ Yes _____

Will you create a care plan? ○ No ○ Yes _____

Does your agency provide in writing the care services provided and clearly describe all rates and fees?

○ No ○ Yes _____

Is there a process for updating the services provided if our needs change?

○ No ○ Yes _____

Can your agency provide 24-hour care? ○ No ○ Yes _____

Does your agency provide transportation services for clients?

○ No ○ Yes _____

Can your agency provide emergency monitoring systems and other safety technology?

○ No ○ Yes _____

FILLED OUT BY: : DATE:

Questions About Certifications and Liability

What are your education and training requirements for caregivers?

Is your agency licensed or accredited by any government agency to provide home care? Is your agency Medicare-certified?

O No O Yes

Do you carry liability insurance?

O No O Yes

Are your employees bonded and insured for theft and client injury?

O No O Yes

Do you perform background checks on employees?

O No O Yes

Can your agency provide documentation explaining the client's rights, your code of ethics, workers' compensation and HIPAA compliance?

O No O Yes

Do you pay your federal and state taxes, Social Security (FICA) and unemployment insurance so that our family is not legally responsible?

O No O Yes

Can you verify that you and your employees are legally able to work in the United States?

O No O Yes

If your employee is injured at a client's residence, who is responsible?
(Many homeowner's insurance policies exclude injuries to "domestic employees.")

Questions About Working with a Paid Caregiver

Can we meet the person before receiving services?
O No O Yes _____

Do you send the same person each time?
O No O Yes _____

Do you provide back-up coverage in case your employee cannot make it to work?
O No O Yes _____

How do you monitor/supervise employees?
_____

How do you document that your services were indeed completed?
_____

Questions About Administration

Is there someone I can call with questions or complaints?
O No O Yes _____

Can you provide a list of references?
O No O Yes _____

What are the fees for your services (per hour, per day)?
_____

What is the billing schedule for services?
Is there a payment plan option?
O No O Yes _____

Do you require a minimum number of hours per shift? If so, what is it?
O No O Yes _____

How quickly can you initiate service?
_____

CHAPTER SIX

Planning Ahead

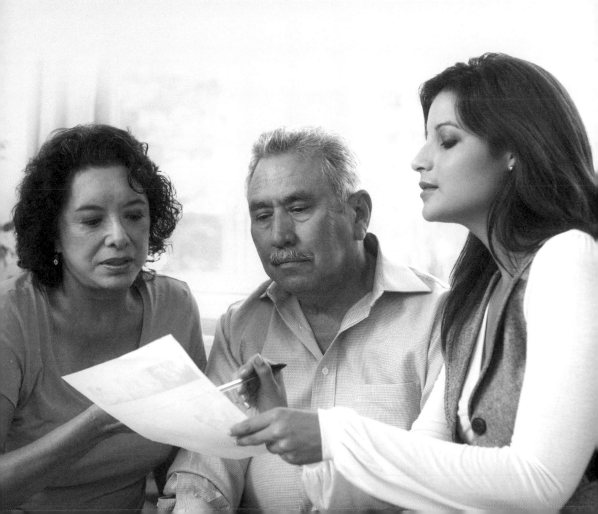

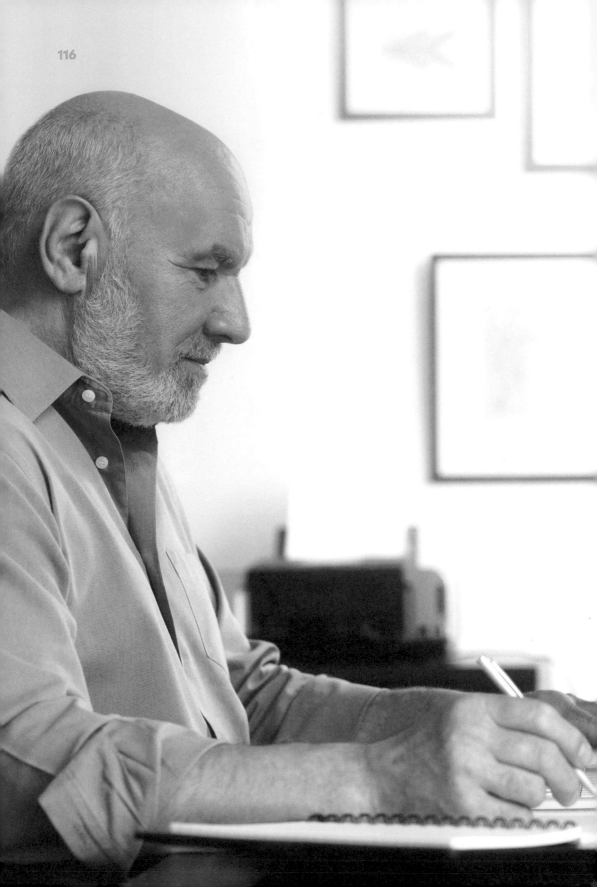

Planning Ahead

There are steps every adult should take, regardless of health status, to align your values, wishes and preferences with medical care you will receive. It is important to take time to develop these plans for both you and your loved one. This section will help you discuss and prepare for the future. Start your planning whenever you and your loved one are ready – the sooner the better.

IN THIS CHAPTER

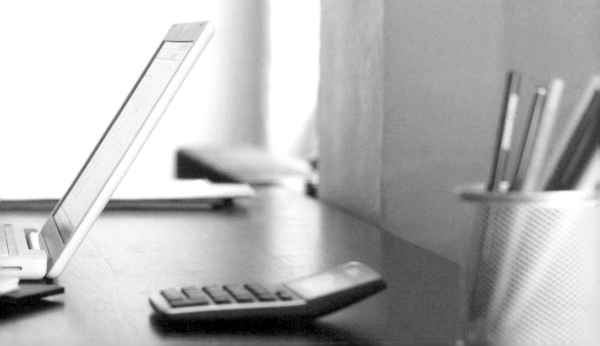

Be Prepared

No one can predict future needs, so it is wise to consider a variety of possible scenarios and be prepared for them.

For example, it can be hard to imagine a time when your loved one will need skilled nursing care or will not be able to make his or her own decisions. However, the best time to plan for these situations is now, before they occur. In fact, many people report a sense of relief and optimism after having the opportunity to share their thoughts and wishes.

Periodically assess your caregiving situation to reevaluate your strengths and weaknesses and identify your personal limits. What areas of providing care are "too much" for you, either emotionally or physically? Who in the family or community can you call upon to supplement the care that you provide? Think about how long you will be able to care for the person with Parkinson's at home. All of these factors should go into your planning.

I have lived with Parkinson's disease for over 20 years. My wife and I have taken steps to prepare for the future, but we are going to live the day as it is. We take it one step at a time. It's just like driving – look ahead. See what's coming next.

– FREDERICK, DIAGNOSED MORE THAN 20 YEARS AGO

Maintaining Important Information

It is important to keep an up-to-date record of your loved one's medical information and medical history that can be accessed by first responders in case of an emergency. In fact, you should create such a record for yourself, as well.

Keep these lists updated and in a location that is easily visible and accessible in an emergency. Make sure friends and family know the location. Some people keep this list near their medications, as emergency personnel will often seek these out if called to your home.

Information to include:

- Date information was last updated
- Name, address, phone number and date of birth
- Current medications (both prescription and over-the-counter), with prescribing physician, purpose, dosage and frequency
- Primary and specialty care physicians and contact information
- Allergies
- Medical conditions
- Surgeries (and year)
- Blood type
- Advance directives
- Two emergency contacts (name, phone)

Advance Care Planning

Advance care planning allows you and your loved one to state your wishes about future healthcare treatments and to designate a person to represent your wishes in the event you become incapable of expressing those wishes or choose to delegate decision-making.

It is recommended that all adults create an advance directive. Social workers, elder law attorneys or other specially trained staff or community volunteers can assist in this process. Completed documents should be shared with your physician, local hospital and family members.

Advance Directive for Healthcare

HEALTHCARE DECLARATION, DIRECTIVE TO PHYSICIANS, LIVING WILL

- Allows you to put into writing your wishes about medical treatment should you have a terminal condition and be unable to communicate.
- May include specific directions about death-delaying procedures you do or do not want (e.g., artificial life support, transfusions, dialysis).
- "Terminal illness" means incurable or irreversible, where death is imminent.
- Regulations for witnesses and notary vary by state.

Durable Power of Attorney for Healthcare

MEDICAL POWER OF ATTORNEY, HEALTHCARE PROXY

- Names a healthcare agent to make decisions that reflect your wishes, if/when you are unable to make your own decisions.
- Agent must be a legal adult who is required to speak according to your specific instructions.
- If agent is unsure of your wishes in a specific situation, the agent is required to speak in your "best interest."
- Names alternate or successor agents who serve one at a time, in order (sometimes called surrogate decision makers).
- Regulations (e.g., notary) vary by state, but every state recognizes Durable Power of Attorney for Healthcare.
- Should be periodically reviewed, re-dated and initialed.
- Can be ended at any time by informing doctor and agent and destroying the document.

- Contains instructions related to the following:
  - Life-support measures: Various measures can be used to replace or enhance a failing body function. These can be used temporarily until illness is stabilized and the body can resume normal functioning, but these measures can also prolong the dying process and diminish quality of life.
    - Several types of tube feeding can sustain life.
      See "End of Life Planning" on page 169, in the "Advanced Parkinson's" section, for more information on artificial nutrition and hydration.
    - A mechanical ventilation respirator or ventilator supplies oxygen to support or replace impaired lung function.
    - Cardiopulmonary resuscitation (CPR) is an emergency lifesaving procedure that is done when someone's breathing or heartbeat has stopped.
  - Anatomical (organ) donation
  - Disposal of remains

POLST (Physician Orders for Life-Sustaining Treatment)

There is a document increasingly being used in addition to the healthcare power of attorney. The POLST (Physician Orders for Life-Sustaining Treatment) is a signed medical order that communicates patient preferences to healthcare providers during an emergency.
It is recommended for people with complicated medical problems who have limited life expectancy or would like to set limits on care received.
Refer to "End of Life Planning" on page 169, in the "Advanced Parkinson's" section, for more information on POLST.

Do Not Resuscitate ("No Code")

- Doctor's written order instructing nursing and hospital staff that, if a person's heart or breathing stops, the person does not wish to be revived (i.e., to receive CPR).
- May specify means by which person would or would not want to be revived: mouth-to-mouth, pressing on chest, electric shock, drugs.
- Requires the following to be in effect:
  - Patient consent and signature
  - Witnesses
  - Physician's signature
  - Inclusion in patient's medical record

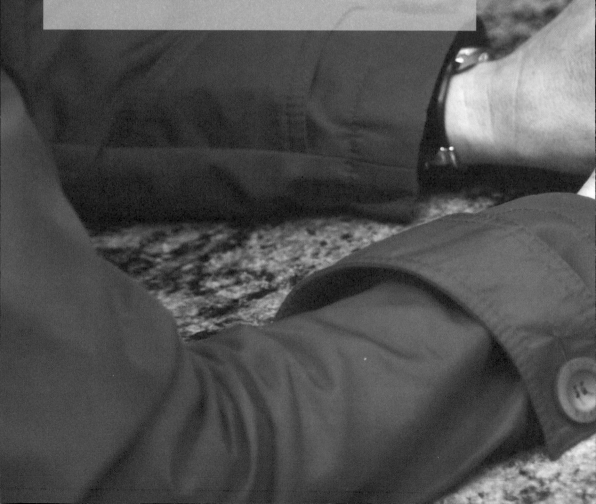

CARING MOMENT

Talk about your wishes for the future.

Sharing can be difficult, but it has both practical and emotional benefits.

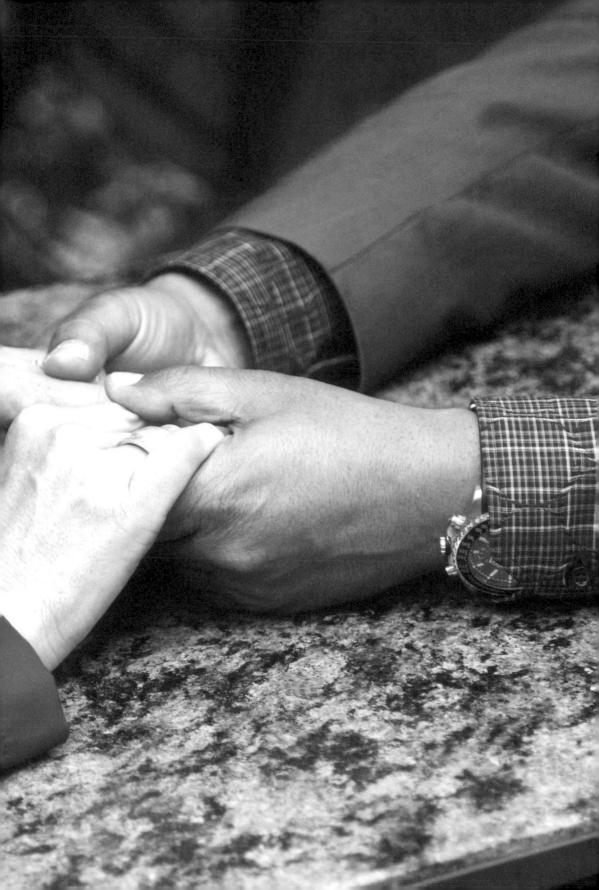

Is a Care Facility Needed?

People with advancing Parkinson's require safe and effective care, all the time. The day may come when this level of care cannot be provided at home. If this day comes, you should consider a transition to a more supportive living environment.

There are certainly benefits to keeping the person with Parkinson's at home. The environment is familiar (and comforting), and you won't have to travel to see him or her. Despite the challenges of caregiving, the relationship between you and the person with Parkinson's often becomes stronger over time. There can also be considerable savings in healthcare costs.

On the other hand, as the disease progresses and the person's needs become more extreme, keeping the person at home can seem like a battle of your survival versus his or hers. If you are caring for your loved one in your home, the escalating demands of the disease might negatively impact your relationship with others living in the house.

Tough Decisions

Undoubtedly, making the decision to move your loved one out of the home is an emotional process. People have called it "the hardest decision of my life." Be prepared for potential accusations of abandonment and your own feelings of guilt. Other family members living out of town or not providing direct care may disagree with your decision. A family meeting facilitated by a neutral professional such as a social worker or geriatric care manager may help get everyone on the same page and make the transition easier.

Hopefully the following fact will help you and the person with Parkinson's overcome any negative emotions: **the move to a care facility does not negate your role as caregiver**. Many family caregivers spend a lot of time at the care facility after the transition. You will need to explain Parkinson's disease to the facility staff and constantly advocate for your loved one's needs.

The person with Parkinson's may enjoy the potential benefits of a care facility:
• Increased access to social activities offered at the residence
• Opportunities for involvement by on-site medical and rehab professionals
• A more accessible environment
• Available staff to provide assistance at all hours of the day and night

How do I know if home care is possible?

As Parkinson's progresses and your loved one's needs increase, the following factors must be considered when determining whether home care will work for you:

- **The designated caregiver should have few other responsibilities** not related to the person with Parkinson's: if you have a job, it will be difficult to provide comprehensive home care. If the designated caregiver is someone you hire to provide around-the-clock care, consider the impact of someone else living in your home. Even though you are not responsible for daily caregiving chores, having another person in your house might cause stress and make it difficult to relax in your own home.

- **The house must be large enough** to comfortably accommodate the needs of the person with Parkinson's, including space for a walker, wheelchair, bedside commode or other medical equipment required.

- **All rooms should be on one level.** The home environment must be safe and supportive of maximum independence. Necessary structural changes, such as ramps, handrails, bathroom alterations, etc. have been made.

- **Arrangements can be made to provide medications** to the person with Parkinson's at required times, as well as meals, assistance with personal care, housekeeping, transportation and companionship.

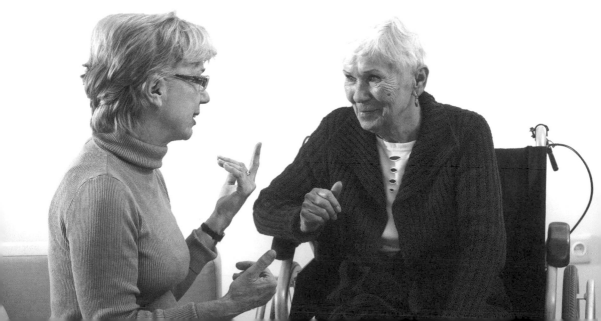

- **Financial considerations do not permit it** (e.g., when the family caregiver must maintain other employment). Many people believe that Medicare will pay for in-home care, but there are strict eligibility requirements (a person must be essentially homebound and need intermittent skilled care).

- **Family limitations do not permit it** (time, space, young children still at home).

- **Caregiver's physical and emotional strength is depleted.**

- **Patient's condition** requires skilled nursing care or round-the-clock attention.

- **The patient is a "two person assist,"** requiring two people to get him or her out of bed, out of a chair, off the toilet, etc.

- **Physical layout of the home** is unsuitable.

- **Person with Parkinson's prefers to live independent of family.**

Be Prepared

It is a good idea to visit a few facilities before a transition is necessary to get an idea of the available choices. It will allow you time to make the decision and will be less stressful than "starting cold" following a hospital stay and discharge necessitating finding a place on short notice. Take a friend or geriatric care manager with you to help assess the services and environment. You might also want to familiarize yourself with palliative (comfort) care options, including hospice, so that if the need arises you will know where to turn.

See "Palliative and Hospice Care" on page 172, in the "Advanced Parkinson's" section, for more information.

Types of Care Facilities

If considering a move from the home environment, it is important to understand the wide variety of options providing long-term care. Long-term care facilities are on a spectrum from most to least independent living.

INDEPENDENT LIVING

These types of buildings are not licensed to provide personal care or nursing services, although residents can and do contract for private duty care just as they would in their own home or apartment (*see the tip sheet "Action Plan for Hiring In-Home Caregivers" on page 90*). All of these more independent facilities offer amenities such as 24-hour security, transportation and activity programs. Whereas senior apartments and active communities may not serve meals in a central dining room, retirement homes usually do have group dining.

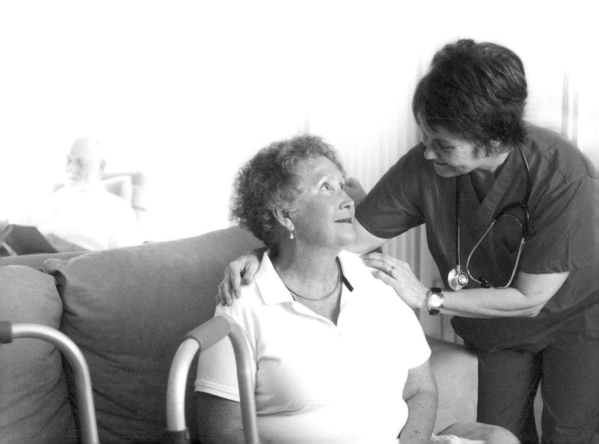

ASSISTED LIVING

An assisted living facility can provide supervision and assistance with care as needed. It is designed for situations when independent living is not appropriate, but 24-hour nursing home care is not needed. Caregivers are nurses or trained, certified aides who assist with daily tasks such as bathing, dressing, escort to meals, medication set-up and dispensing and routine checks on residents. Fees for these personal and nursing cares vary by facility. Assisted living facilities also provide housekeeping and social programs, as well as transportation to and from medical appointments, errands and group outings. Some facilities may offer rehabilitation therapies, hospice care and specialized care for different disorders.

CONTINUING CARE RETIREMENT COMMUNITIES

Continuing care retirement communities (CCRCs) are residential, gate-secured campuses that, with a substantial entrance fee, guarantee lifelong care beginning with independent living (cottages or apartments) and progressing to assisted living and then skilled (nursing home) care.

NURSING HOMES

Nursing homes are facilities that are licensed and regulated by state and federal governments to provide skilled care 24 hours a day. Registered nurses are on-duty round-the-clock, as are certified nurses' aides. Physicians serve as medical directors of skilled care facilities. Everything from activities to nutrition, personal care, environmental safety and staff-to-resident ratios must meet state and federal guidelines.

CHAPTER SEVEN

Advanced
Parkinson's

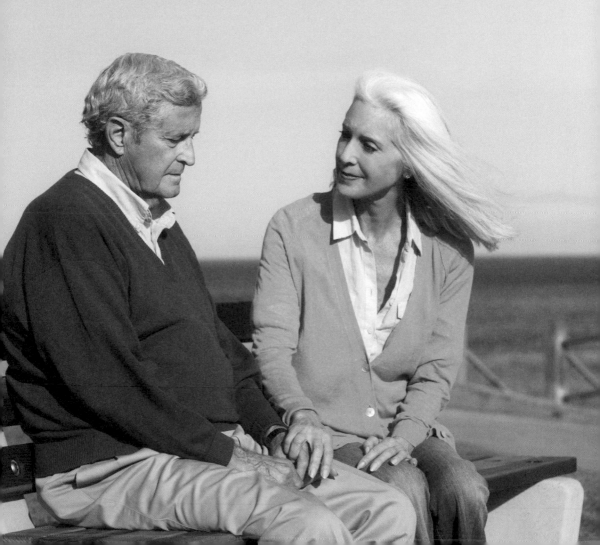

Advanced Parkinson's

Despite the challenges of advanced Parkinson's, there is still a lot you can do to make life easier and more enjoyable both for yourself and your loved one. The following pages provide tips and resources to help you provide the best possible care for your loved one with advanced-stage Parkinson's. The information may also be helpful to professional caregivers who work with your loved one in the home environment.

IN THIS CHAPTER

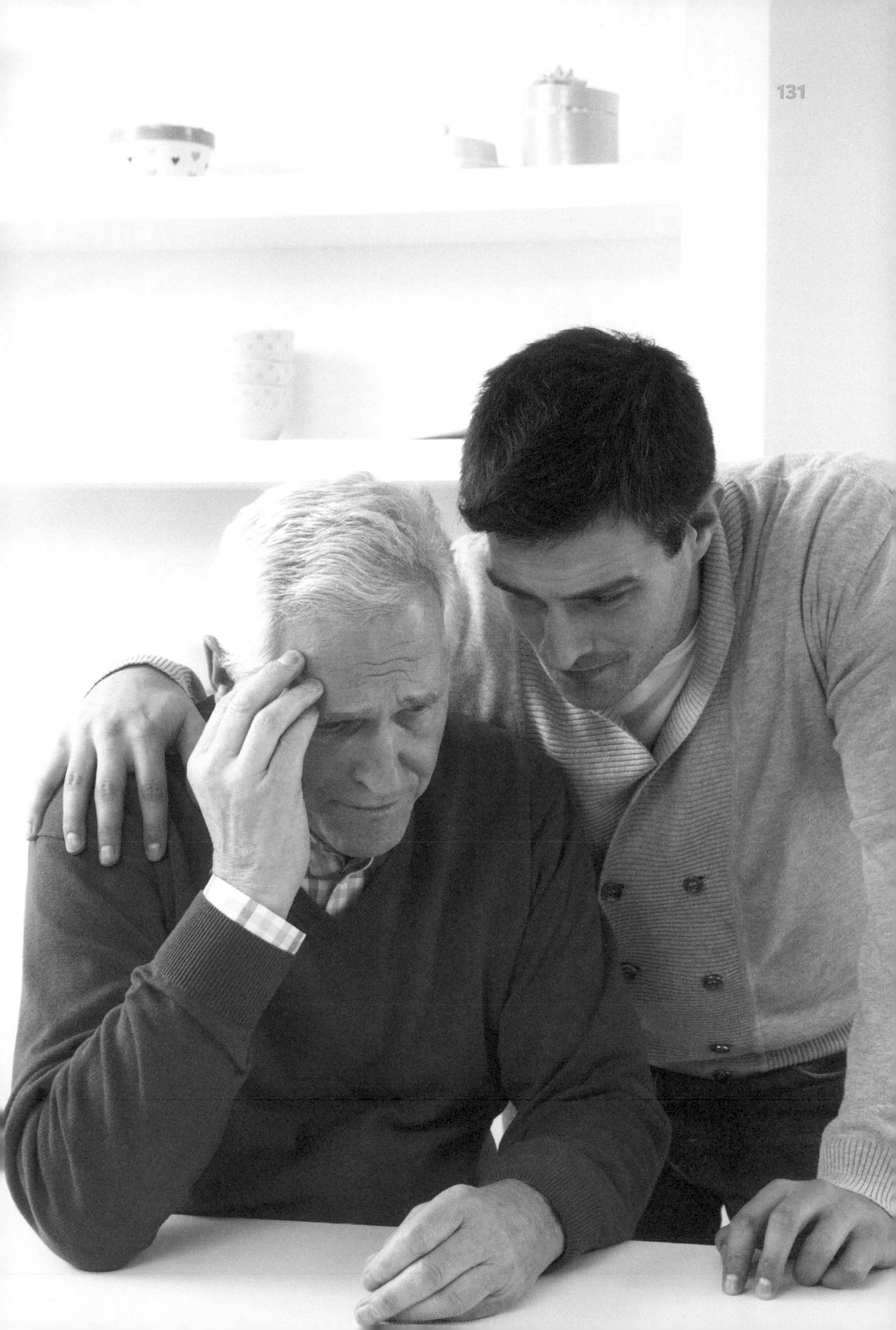

What Is Advanced Parkinson's?

There is no one definition of what it means to have "advanced" Parkinson's disease. Everyone is unique, and the disease progresses differently from person to person. However, there are several scales used in research and by healthcare providers to measure how severe the disease is and how far it has progressed. In general, when a person with Parkinson's is no longer physically independent, the disease is considered advanced.

This means that the person has serious problems with mobility and cannot complete activities of daily living by himself or herself. Cognition changes – specifically dementia – are also a hallmark of advanced PD.

Each person with Parkinson's is unique, so the suggestions in this chapter may need to be modified for your particular situation. You are strongly recommended to seek and build a team of professionals in your local area to help you on your caregiving journey.

If you need help locating providers, call the Parkinson's Foundation Helpline at **1-800-4PD-INFO** (473-4636).

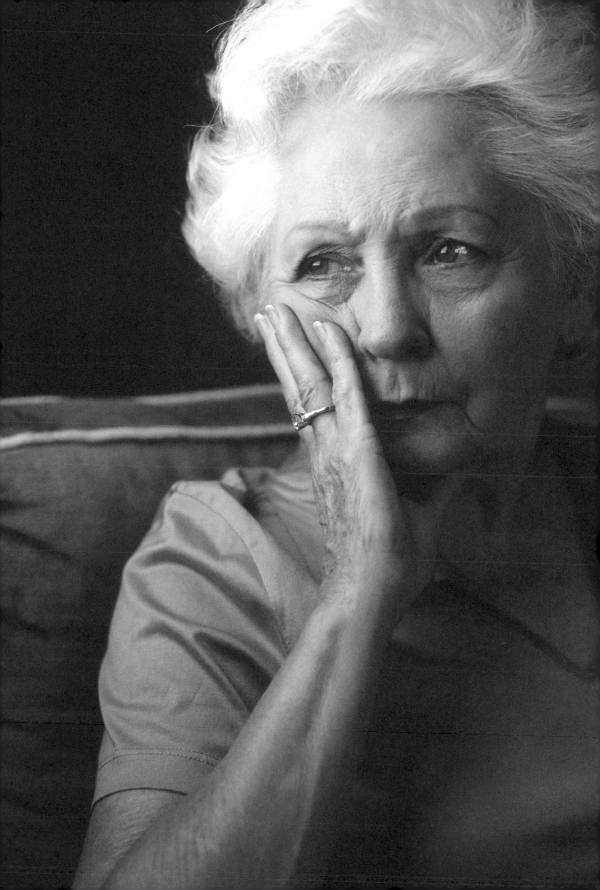

TIP SHEET

Plans and Scheduling

Caregivers are busy! But you already know that. Being organized and establishing a daily routine will help you save time and energy.

General Tips

» **Prioritize** what needs to be done each day.

» **Try to stick to a daily routine.** Your loved one will usually function better if he or she knows what is going to happen each day.

» **Use a calendar or day planner** to record appointments and activities.

» **Maintain a shopping list** to organize errands or quickly ask others to provide help.

» **Cluster items together in a bin**, so you can easily gather everything when providing care to the person with Parkinson's.

» **Try to make time with your loved one that is not focused on caregiving tasks.**

» **Schedule time to rest** within the daily routine.

» **Investigate options for home delivery** of groceries, medications and household supplies.

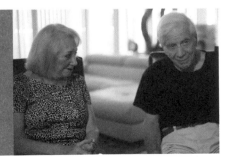

WATCH THE VIDEOS

Plans and Scheduling, Parts 1 and 2

Online at Parkinson.org/videos in the "CareMAP How-to Videos" playlist

Recording Important Information

» **Keep important names and phone numbers on an updated contact list.**
Post this list in a visible area. *(See "Contact List" worksheet on page 8.)*

» **Keep paper and pens next to the phone** to record messages or numbers.

» **Write down the daily routine** so it can be done by others if you are unable.
See "Daily Routine" worksheet on page 104.

» **Create and maintain a list of your loved one's medications**
with dosage, timing and frequency.
See "Medications and Schedule" worksheet on page 64.

» **Keep accurate records of financial and insurance information.**

» **Review your loved one's advance healthcare directive** to ensure the
named healthcare agent and wishes are current.
See "Advance Care Planning" on page 120 in the "Planning Ahead" section.

» **Make sure a trusted family member or friend knows the location of
important information.**

Exploring Care Options
Think about the "what if" scenarios: what if your loved one becomes ill,
you become ill or you both become ill? Set up a plan, and discuss the plan
with family and friends.

» **Consult a social worker or geriatric case manager** to learn about
programs, services and care options appropriate for both current
and future needs.

» **Talk with members of your support group** to learn about possible options.

» **Make sure you understand benefits and covered services** included in your
current insurance plan, including any long-term care policies.

» **Investigate options for home care, adult day services, respite stays,
assisted living or long-term care in your area.** Keep this information
available as needed.

» **Tour care facilities in advance of need** to prevent last minute decisions.
Your preferred facility may have a waiting list.

Movement Challenges

It is essential to address your loved one's physical and mobility challenges. As Parkinson's progresses, you will likely need to provide greater hands-on assistance and learn safe and effective ways to provide help without injuring yourself or the person with Parkinson's. Talk to your loved one's healthcare provider to obtain a referral to a physical therapist (PT). PTs are trained to provide an evaluation and assist you in developing the best methods for your situation.

Standing and Sitting

When at home, make sure that your loved one uses a chair with sturdy arm rests and a stable sitting base. Avoid soft, low seating or upholstery such as velour or velvet, which can make movements more difficult to perform. You can also raise seat height by adding an extra cushion to the chair or using a sturdy folded blanket.

» When attempting to get up, make sure the person with Parkinson's first **scoots his hips forward to the edge of the chair**.

» Make sure your loved one's **feet are placed firmly underneath him before standing**. You may need to help with proper foot placement.

» **Use cues like "nose over toes"** to give the person with Parkinson's a goal for leaning forward, easing the transfer out of a chair.

» When helping the person with Parkinson's stand up, **avoid pulling on his arms or legs as he tries to stand**.

» A **transfer belt** often makes providing assistance safer and easier. (These belts can be purchased at a medical equipment store.)

» Make sure the person with Parkinson's puts **both hands on the arm rests and leans forward** as he tries to sit down. Remind him to wait until he feels the chair against the backs of both legs before attempting to sit. This helps maintain smooth, controlled motion and avoids "crash landings," which can be dangerous and hard on the person's spine.

» If the person with Parkinson's uses a walker, make sure he continues to use this device as he turns to sit down.

If the person with Parkinson's is no longer able to provide assistance getting up and down with hands on arm rests, it may be best to stand directly in front of him, grasping the transfer belt with both hands. Using a pre-arranged count or signal, assist the person to his feet, then slowly perform a pivot turn in the direction of the wheelchair or other surface he is moving to. *(For a demonstration, watch the video "Movement and Falls Part 1" in the "CareMAP: How-to Videos" playlist at Parkinson.org/videos.)*

Walking

Walking changes are common in Parkinson's disease and can become more difficult to manage as PD progresses. People with Parkinson's often need reminders, or "cues," to take long steps as automatic motions become more difficult to perform.

» **Avoid distractions when walking**. Attempts to do more than one thing at the same time make walking and balance more difficult.

» **Focus on the size of the steps.** Larger steps make walking more stable.

» **Keep your instructions and cues short and simple**, e.g., "Big steps."

» To help with increasing pace (called festination), **provide a cue** to stop then start over with big steps.

» **Freezing** (feet glued to floor) is a significant cause of falls.

  – Freezing often happens while turning around in close quarters. Try to avoid tight turns whenever possible. Instruct your loved one to make wider turns.

  – To help with freezing, count or clap a rhythmic beat.

  – Some people who experience freezing episodes do better with a visual cue, such as "step over my foot."

» If the person with Parkinson's has a tendency to lose his balance backward, **position yourself slightly behind the person** as he stands and walks to help minimize this problem.

» **Watch out for pets** in the home!

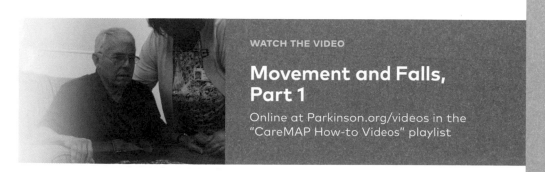

WATCH THE VIDEO

Movement and Falls, Part 1

Online at Parkinson.org/videos in the "CareMAP How-to Videos" playlist

Walking with Assistive Devices

Your loved one's physical therapist can help determine if an assistive device is necessary and what kind will be most effective.

» The assistive device must be **fitted by a professional** to ensure safe and effective use.

» **Avoid four-post walkers or quad canes**, which can be difficult for the person with Parkinson's to move effectively. A walker with wheels may work best.

» **The physical therapist can help you get the right assistive device** in the best method for insurance reimbursement.

Wheelchair

If mobility changes do not allow the person with Parkinson's to walk, a wheelchair may be necessary. There are many wheelchair options.

» **Consult with a rehab therapist** or other provider who can make a full assessment of the type of chair needed and fit it to ensure your loved one's best posture, positioning and comfort.

» **Always lock the brakes** so the chair is stable and does not move as the person gets up or down.

» **Make sure the wheelchair fits** through your home's doorways, into the bathroom or anywhere else needed to provide care throughout the day.

It is sometimes hard for Eleanor and me to remember to focus on her walking. We tend to want to continue our conversations, but we have learned she has much more success if we stop talking and think about the task at hand.

– DON, CARES FOR ELEANOR

Getting Up from a Fall

Even with safety precautions in place, sometimes falls occur. It is important to have a back-up plan before a fall happens. Do you have a friend, relative or neighbor who is able to help? Do you need an emergency call button or other system installed in your home to summon help? Know the process to activate an emergency call if needed.

It is also important to learn a safe method for helping the person up from the ground to avoid injury to both you and the person with Parkinson's. Work with a physical therapist to prepare a system in case a fall occurs.

» **Don't panic!**

» Take time to **make sure the person is not injured and has an opportunity to rest** if needed before trying to get up. Poor planning can result in a second fall.

» **Have the person with Parkinson's scoot to a solid piece of furniture** or another object that she can use to help pull herself up.

» A **transfer belt** can provide you with a firm grip to aid the person as she rises. Work together and make sure everyone is aware of the plan before starting to get up.

» If you determine that it is unsafe to help the person up without more assistance, **call for help**. As you wait for help to arrive, make the person with Parkinson's as comfortable as possible.

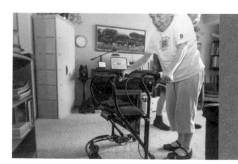

WATCH THE VIDEO

Movement and Falls, Part 2

Online at Parkinson.org/videos in the "CareMAP How-to Videos" playlist

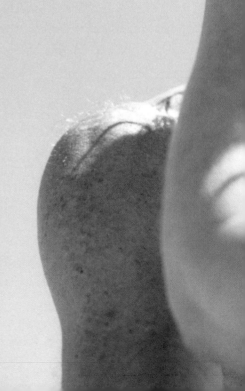

CARING MOMENT

Be present in every moment.

Give each activity with the person with Parkinson's – a conversation, a movement, a caring task – your full attention.

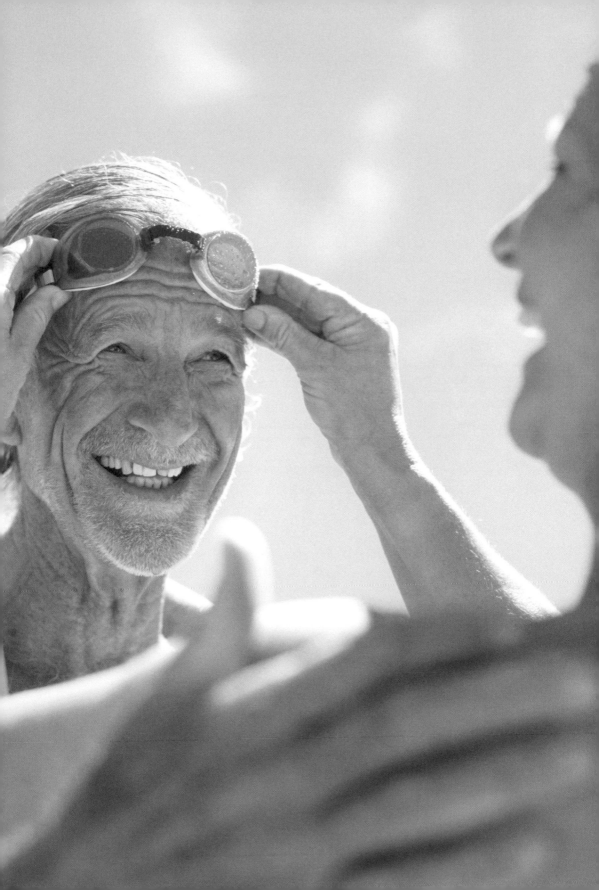

Dressing

Advancing Parkinson's can make daily tasks more difficult to perform. Getting dressed becomes a slower, more challenging activity, and caregivers often need to provide assistance. Changes to clothing and the dressing routine can improve safety and reduce frustration.

General Tips

» **Ensure adequate time for dressing.** Stress can make PD symptoms worse, so your loved one may not be able to help as much if you are rushing.

» Consider **waiting for a time to dress** when your loved one's PD medications are working well, and he or she has the best mobility possible.

» **Assemble all necessary clothing items before beginning** to dress to eliminate multiple trips to the closet or dresser.

» Allow the person with Parkinson's to **provide as much assistance as he or she can**.

» **Offer choice** (red sweater or blue sweater?) and encourage participation in physical movement.

» **Incorporate a few extra arm or leg motions** for the person with Parkinson's during dressing to keep muscles flexible. This also builds range of motion and flexibility exercise into the daily routine.

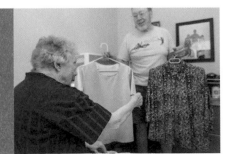

WATCH THE VIDEO

Dressing
Online at Parkinson.org/videos in the "CareMAP How-to Videos" playlist

Staying Safe While Dressing

» Have the person with Parkinson's **sit down while dressing** to reduce the risk of balance loss or falls.

» To reduce back strain, make sure you have the **best positioning possible** when helping the person with Parkinson's get dressed. For example, you can put on his or her pants, socks and shoes while the person is still lying down.

What to Wear?

» **Choose clothing styles and fabrics that make dressing easier.**

» Select clothes that are **easy to put on.**

    – Soft, stretchy fabrics are better if stiffness and rigidity are a problem.

    – Elastic waistbands, front openings and bras that hook in front are good choices.

    – Tube socks may be easier to put on than dress socks.

» **Avoid velour and similar fabrics**, which can create more friction with other surfaces and make it difficult to dress or move during the day.

» If one arm or leg has more stiffness, put this extremity into the sleeve or pant leg **first**.

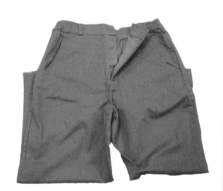

» **Velcro can be sewn into existing clothes** (replace buttons with Velcro closures). Or you can buy clothing designed for easier dressing from adaptive clothing catalogs.

» **Shoes with Velcro closures** can also make dressing easier.

COLD WEATHER CLIMATES

» Choose outerwear that is **oversized and easy fitting**.

» **A soft fabric coat or sweatshirt** may be easier to put on, or consider an overhead poncho-style coat that does not require fitting arms into sleeves.

» **Mittens** are easier to put on than individual finger gloves.

Mealtime and Swallowing

Advancing Parkinson's frequently causes difficulty with eating and drinking because of both movement and swallowing problems. You might need to change the types of foods you serve or the utensils the person with Parkinson's uses, and you might need to help your loved one eat so he or she gets adequate nutrition.

General Tips

» **Schedule mealtimes when Parkinson's medications are working best.**

» **Use adaptive utensils and cups**, including curved and/or built-up forks and spoons, rocker knives, plate guards, nosey cups and covered cups.

» **An occupational therapist** can help determine what types of adaptive equipment might work best. Ask the doctor for a referral.

» When providing feeding assistance, **give small bites**, and allow adequate time for thorough chewing and a complete swallow.

» Dehydration can occur due to inadequate fluid intake. Know the symptoms: increased confusion, low blood pressure, dizziness, dark colored urine.

Mealtime Set-up

» **Choose a pleasant, quiet environment** without a lot of distractions.

» **Use small pillows or cushions** to keep posture upright.

» **Place the plate and cup on an elevated tray** if your loved one has neck immobility or vision changes.

» **Protect clothing** with a neck napkin, apron or other protective garment.

» Changes in vision may make it more difficult for your loved one if the color of the food is the same color as the dish. **Consider using dark dishes when serving light-colored foods, and light dishes when serving dark foods.**

» **Cut food into bite-size portions.**

Types of Foods to Serve

» **Avoid tough, dry or crumbly textures** that might be difficult to swallow.

» **Consider foods that can be cut into smaller "finger food" portions** to maximize independence.

» **Choose foods that are easier to chew and swallow.** For example:
    – Lean hamburger or beef stew (avoid steak)
    – Baked or broiled fish
    – Eggs (a good way to get protein, and there are many ways to serve them)
    – Cooked vegetables
    – Soft fruits such as berries and melons
    – Rice, whole grains and beans
    – Gravies, sauces or butter (moisten foods for easier swallowing)

» If weight loss is a problem, see "Tips for Gaining Weight" on the next page.

Drinking

» **Make sure your loved one gets 48-64 ounces of liquid daily.** This means 6 to 8 glasses of liquid per day. One easy way to increase daily liquid intake is to drink a glass of water with each Parkinson's medication dose.

» **Encourage sips of liquid between solid foods.**

» **Shorten the length of straws** by cutting off part of the bottom to decrease the volume of liquid consumed through the straw at one time.

» **Serve foods with higher liquid contents**, such as fruits, vegetables, Jell-O and ice cream.

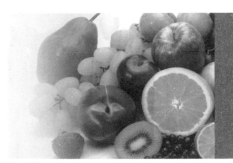

WATCH THE VIDEOS

Mealtime and Swallowing, Parts 1 and 2

Online at Parkinson.org/videos in the "CareMAP How-to Videos" playlist

Mealtime Fatigue

» **Serve small, frequent meals** if your loved one experiences weight loss, low blood pressure or fatigue or feels full quickly.

» **Maintain an upright sitting posture for 30 minutes after each meal** to prevent aspiration.

» **Always give food or medications when your loved one is seated in an upright position**, not when reclined or lying down.

Swallowing Difficulty

» **Report swallowing difficulties**, coughing or choking episodes to the doctor for evaluation.

» **Consider a referral to a speech language pathologist** for evaluation and recommendations for changing food and liquid consistencies for safer swallowing.

» Attend a Red Cross class to **learn the Heimlich maneuver** to be ready in case of an emergency.

» **Feeding tubes** may be considered for those with severe swallowing problems. This is a choice that should be carefully considered with input from the person with Parkinson's, family and the healthcare team.

» Consult your doctor, nurse or pharmacist if whole medications are not able to be swallowed. *See tip sheet "Medications On Time, Every Time" on page 154 for more information.*

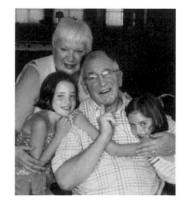

Sometimes we found it was easier to celebrate an occasion without food and not make that the focus. So we would have a birthday party for the kids in a park and have cake and ice cream, and it worked great. We had to shift our thinking a little bit but still have the celebration.

– LENNORE, CARED FOR HUSBAND, ROGER

TIPS FOR GAINING WEIGHT

Weight loss may occur with advancing Parkinson's. Difficulty swallowing, feeling full or bloated and improperly-fitting partial plates or dentures are all potential reasons. Discuss concerns regarding weight loss with your loved one's medical team.

Switch from 3 regular meals to **5-6 smaller meals daily**.

Switch to a higher fat milk, such as 2% or whole milk. Choose flavored milk or whole milk yogurt for variety.

Drink 100% fruit juices instead of water.

Add butter, nut butters, gravy, sauces and/or avocado to the diet to **add calories**.

Eat fruit canned in syrup or frozen with sugar.

Serve vegetables with cheese spreads, sour cream, dips, salad dressings or sauces.

Drink a high calorie nutritional beverage between meals. Even 4 ounces twice daily will add calories.

Choose drink supplements that are high-calorie, not high-protein.

Purchase or blend a nutritional smoothie, using bottled or powder supplements, adding fruit or syrups for flavor.

Blend a milkshake using 2% or whole milk with fresh fruit or syrup and a scoop of ice cream.

Prepare pudding with 2% or whole milk, and top with crushed graham crackers and whipped cream.

Offer ice cream or frozen yogurt, topped with syrup or fruit.

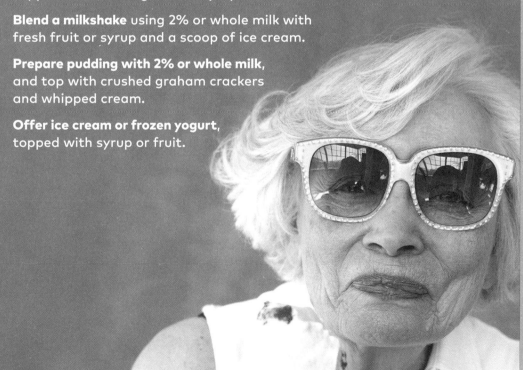

Bathroom

Bathing, toileting, personal hygiene and grooming are basic activities of daily living that advancing Parkinson's makes more challenging. The following tips will help make these activities easier.

Using the Toilet

» Bladder changes in Parkinson's may create the need to use the toilet more frequently, so **create a regular toileting schedule** to help decrease accidents during the day.

» **Limit fluid intake during the evening hours** if the person with Parkinson's has difficulty getting up at night. (It is still important to have adequate fluid intake during the day to prevent dehydration and manage constipation.)

» **Use a stool softener** such as Miralax (recommended by the American Academy of Neurology for treating constipation in PD) to help produce more regular bowel movements. Avoid bulk fiber laxatives, as these require significant fluid consumption to work properly.

» **Install an elevated toilet or place an elevated seat on the existing toilet** to make getting on and off the toilet easier. Some elevated seats have sturdy arm rests attached, or a grab bar can be installed on the wall next to the toilet. This can be helpful to hold onto before pivoting to sit down, or to hold when standing up during the process of hygiene/wiping and clothing adjustment.

» **Make sure your loved one gets close enough to the toilet seat with body properly aligned before attempting to sit down.** Marking the floor with colored tape may help to signal proper foot placement during the transfer.

» **Have moist, flushable hygiene wipes available** in addition to toilet paper to achieve proper cleaning after toileting.

» **Make sure the person with Parkinson's is able to wash his or her hands**, even if this needs to be accomplished from a seated position.

» **Consider buying incontinence pads** if the person with Parkinson's has accidents during the day. Larger pads can be placed on the bed if incontinence is a problem at night. Read pad labels and packaging carefully to determine proper sizing.

Bathing

» **Make sure the room is warm, and gather all necessary supplies before you turn on the water.**

» **Use a walk-in shower with handheld nozzle**, grab bar and tub bench with a back rest when possible for safe bathing.

» **Consider a tub bench that extends over the side of the tub** if a bathtub is the only available option.

» **Use a non-slip mat** to decrease falls risk.

» **Adjust the water temperature before the person with Parkinson's enters the bath.** Use warm water and gentle water pressure.

» **Rinse skin and hair well.**

» **Wrap your loved one in a robe or towel after bathing.** Make sure skin is dried thoroughly. Powders and lotions should be used to ensure good skin care.

» **Consider a bed bath** if immobility prevents getting into a tub or shower. Make sure the water is warm and the person is covered to only expose the portion of the body being washed and dried. Raise bed height if possible to ensure good caregiver body mechanics.

» **Use hand sanitizer gels, antibacterial soaps and moist towelettes throughout the day to maintain hygiene.**

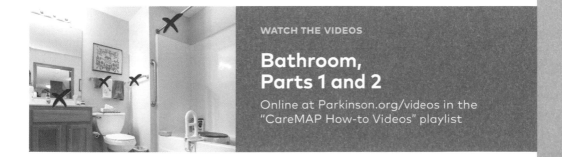

WATCH THE VIDEOS

Bathroom, Parts 1 and 2

Online at Parkinson.org/videos in the "CareMAP How-to Videos" playlist

Shaving

» **Use an electric razor.**

» **Rinse the skin well** with a wet washcloth and pat dry. Apply a soothing lotion; aftershave astringents are often too harsh for older skin.

Oral Care

» **Assemble needed supplies in advance** (soft toothbrush, fluoride toothpaste, small basin for rinsing, dental floss picks). An electric or sonic toothbrush may be used to promote better oral health.

» **Choose a place that is comfortable.**
The kitchen or dining room may be better than the bathroom.

» **Make sure you have good light.**
Sit or stand where you can see all surfaces of the teeth.

» **Brush your loved one's teeth twice daily.**
Be patient and verbalize each step in the process.

» **Keep a small towel nearby for quick clean-up.**

» **Rinse with a mouthwash that does not contain alcohol.**
Use oral swabs (small sponges on a stick) soaked in mouthwash between meals to clean and freshen the mouth.

It is hard for Walter to stand at the bathroom sink. So we set up for brushing teeth while seated at the kitchen table. He uses his shaving mirror, a small basin, and a glass of water. I bring his electric toothbrush and paste to the table. A regular electric toothbrush was hard to handle because of its size and weight. We use a child-size electric toothbrush for better results.

– ALICE, CARES FOR WALTER

Thinking Changes and Dementia

A broad spectrum of potential thinking and memory changes can occur in people with Parkinson's disease, including slowed thought processes, forgetfulness, confusion about routine tasks, lack of judgment, compulsive behaviors, paranoia, anxiety and personality changes.

Some people with advanced Parkinson's disease experience more profound changes in thinking (dementia). It is important to acknowledge and adapt to these changes even though they can be frustrating and frightening for both the person with Parkinson's and the family. Promptly report any new or sudden changes in thinking or behavior to the healthcare team.

General Tips

» **A smile and pleasant manner** can invite cooperation.

» **Speak at eye level and maintain eye contact.**

» **Use the same cues each time to provide instructions.**
Teach these cues to anyone who provides care.

» **Do not leave someone with thinking changes or dementia alone.**
Lack of judgment and/or impulsive behaviors can create a dangerous situation.

» **Try using humor to diffuse a stressful situation, but avoid using negative humor or sarcastic remarks,** which may be misinterpreted.

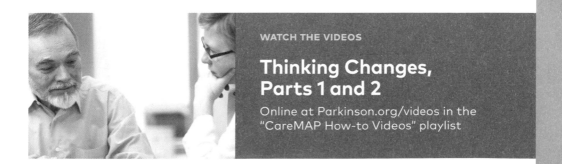

WATCH THE VIDEOS

Thinking Changes, Parts 1 and 2
Online at Parkinson.org/videos in the "CareMAP How-to Videos" playlist

Slowed Thinking

» **Ask one question at a time.**

» **Give the person with Parkinson's time to respond to a question before making an assumption that he or she does not care to answer.**
Try counting to 10 before asking the question again.

» **Ask either/or questions instead of open-ended questions.**
For example, instead of asking, "What do you want to wear today?" ask, "Do you want to wear the red shirt or the blue shirt?"

» **Try giving a one or two word hint** if the person with Parkinson's has difficulty finding a word or loses his or her train of thought.

» **Use short, simple phrases to provide cues.** Avoid using too many words when providing direction.

Forgetfulness and Confusion

» **Cross days off on the calendar.**

» **Keep frequently needed items in a consistent place.**

» **Note the daily schedule or special event for the day on a chalk or white board.** Place a clock near the board as a reference for the written schedule.

» **Use simple remote controls or cover unnecessary buttons** with tape to decrease confusion.

» **Limit distractions as you try to accomplish the daily routine.**
For example, turn off the TV and radio during dressing and eating.

For more information, order your free copy of our book Cognition: A Mind Guide to Parkinson's *by calling our Helpline at 1-800-4PD-INFO (473-4636).*

I think it is so important, with both Parkinson's and Parkinson's with dementia, to try to relive those moments when things were good, things that might put a smile on their face.

– KAREN, CARED FOR FATHER, JOSEPH

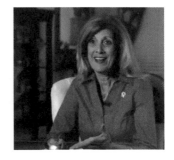

Hallucinations

Hallucinations may occur with disease progression or as a side effect of Parkinson's medications. The term "hallucination" means that someone sees, hears or feels something that is not physically present. It is not a dream or nightmare, but occurs when the person is awake at any time of the day or night. Hallucinations can be bothersome or frightening and should be reported to the medical team.

» **Acknowledge your loved one's experience.** It is ok to say you understand they see something, but you do not see it.

» **Try not to argue** with the person with Parkinson's.

» **Make sure that any medication prescribed for hallucinations is an "atypical antipsychotic"** (does not block dopamine). Check the *Aware in Care* kit for specific information. (Order your free kit and download the resources online at **Parkinson.org/awareincare**).

Behavior and Personality Changes

The person with Parkinson's may experience changes in personality, becoming anxious, moody, irritable or aggressive, even if they were not like this before. Some people develop paranoia (an extreme distrust or suspicion that is not based on reality). At times, they may say or do things that can be hurtful to you as a caregiver. It is extremely difficult to understand and accept this new person. This may cause you to feel sadness, stress, anxiety and depression.

» **Try to avoid confrontations.** It is not usually helpful to try to reason or tell the person with Parkinson's that he or she is wrong.

» **Change the subject or distract the person with Parkinson's with another activity.** It may be helpful to use a familiar activity that represents your loved one's past experiences. For example, an office worker may like to sit at a desk, sort papers, use a calculator or perform other tasks reminiscent of a past life.

» **Try not to get angry or take behavior changes personally.** The person with Parkinson's is not acting out on purpose.

» **Speak in reassuring tones.**

» **Consider what may be causing the behavior.** The person may be hungry, thirsty, tired, in pain, frustrated, lonely or bored.

For more information, order your free copy of our book Psychosis: A Mind Guide to Parkinson's *by calling our Helpline at 1-800-4PD-INFO (473-4636).*

Medications on Time, Every Time

Pills on time is a crucial concept in Parkinson's management. Pills are scheduled at a particular time of day to minimize symptoms as much as possible. Pills given late can lead to greater difficulties for the person with Parkinson's. To make sure your loved one gets his or her medications on schedule, it is necessary to keep everything organized.

General Tips

» **Make sure you keep an updated list** (name, dose, frequency and purpose of the medication; *see "Medications and Schedule" worksheet on page 64 for an easy-to-follow format*). Share this list at each medical appointment.

» **Set up medications in a weekly pill box with a secure lid.**

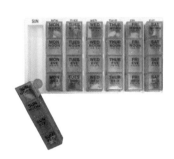

- If medication dosing is 4 times daily or less, you can purchase a weekly pill box with 4 compartments per day. Try to find one with a removable strip for each day, so the day's medications can be easily carried with you when you leave home.

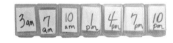

- If dosing is more than 4 times daily, consider purchasing seven weekly pill boxes, using one box for each day. Tape over the days of the week and write down medication dose times.

- Place all medications into pill boxes, including over-the-counter medications.

- Some pharmacies can package medications and will send them to your home on a monthly basis. All medications are organized into individual packets labeled with medication day, date and time to be taken. Check with your pharmacy to see if this is available and if there is a charge for the service. You can also visit www.pillpack.com or call 1-855-745-5725 to arrange for pill delivery.

» **Store all medication bottles and pill boxes in a secure place** where they will not be mistaken for food.

» **Set a reminder for pill times.**
  – A kitchen timer works well at home.
  – When you are out, a cell phone timer or a watch with a vibrating alarm are good options.

» When the alarm sounds indicating pill time, **stop what you are doing and give the medication right away**.

» **When away from home, carry your loved one's daily pills with you.** A long wait at an appointment, heavy traffic or other delay could mean that the next dose is needed before you get home.

» **Check with the Parkinson's doctor before adding new prescriptions or over-the-counter medications** to your loved one's daily schedule. If the person with Parkinson's takes an MAO-B inhibitor (rasagiline, selegiline), some over-the-counter medications may not be safe.

» **Avoid giving multi-symptom over-the-counter medications to your loved one if he or she has a cough or cold.** For example, if the person with Parkinson's has a cough, give medicine for one symptom – the cough – not cough medicine plus decongestant or other ingredient.

» **Do not suddenly stop PD medications for an extended period of time.** For detailed information about the different types of medications used to treat Parkinson's motor and non-motor symptoms, read *Parkinson's Disease: Medications*. You can order a free copy by calling 1-800-4PD-INFO (473-4636) or visiting **Parkinson.org/books**. You can also download the PDF for free.

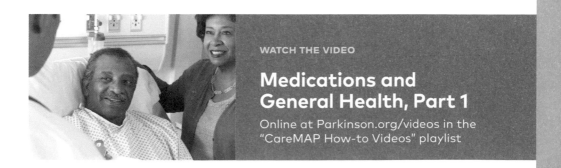

WATCH THE VIDEO

Medications and General Health, Part 1

Online at Parkinson.org/videos in the "CareMAP How-to Videos" playlist

Swallowing Problems

Swallowing changes seen in Parkinson's may result in difficulty taking pills.

» **Offer a sip of water before giving pills.**

» **Provide ample fluid** to reduce swallowing problems and enhance absorption of the medication.

» **Drop pills (whole or crushed) into applesauce for easier swallowing.** Do not crush controlled release or long-acting carbidopa/levodopa or stalevo or entacapone.

» **Avoid giving Parkinson's medications in pudding or ice cream.** The protein in these foods may interfere with Parkinson's medication absorption.

» **Consult your doctor, nurse or pharmacist if the person with Parkinson's cannot swallow whole medications.**

» **There may be options other than a pill for the person with Parkinson's to take carbidopa levodopa.** These include "melt in your mouth" tablets and a levodopa gel delivered directly to the intestines through a pump surgically inserted into the abdomen. The gel method helps prevent levodopa from breaking down and helps the body absorb the levodopa faster, so levodopa levels stay more constant. Ask your loved one's doctor about these options.

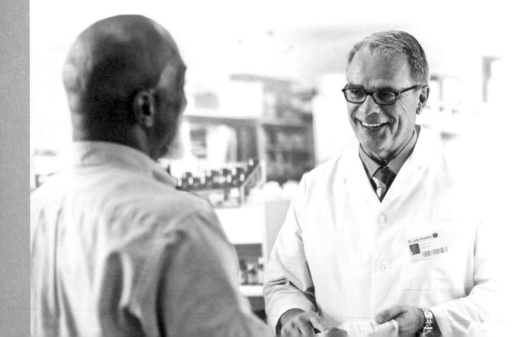

Skin Protection

Parkinson's symptoms can impact the skin. People with Parkinson's have an increased risk of developing melanoma, a type of skin cancer linked to sun exposure. The person with Parkinson's may also have more difficulty changing position, which can result in skin breakdown. Consider these recommendations to protect the skin.

» **Avoid hot, mid-day sun and seek shade when outside.** Make sure the person with Parkinson's uses sunscreen and wears a hat and sunglasses.

» **Help your loved one change position every two hours.** If your loved one is in a wheelchair, get a cushion to lessen the risk of pressure sores. See an occupational or rehab therapist to make sure the right cushions are used.

» **Check skin regularly for redness, blisters and/or open sores.** Report any changes promptly to a member of the medical team.

» **Avoid skin contact with plastic coating and tapes from incontinence products;** these can irritate the skin.

» **Use lotion to prevent dryness.**

» **Consider an eggcrate or alternating pressure mattress pad** to reduce pressure points.

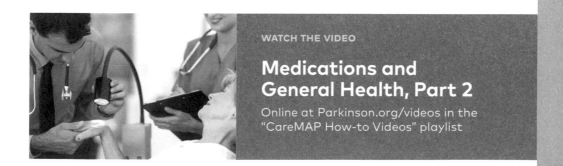

WATCH THE VIDEO

Medications and General Health, Part 2

Online at Parkinson.org/videos in the "CareMAP How-to Videos" playlist

Managing Pain

Pain can be a symptom in Parkinson's, and it can be attributed to many causes. Complaints of pain should be discussed with the doctor. Most people can safely take over-the-counter analgesics to decrease pain. Check with the physician for advice on which pain reliever is best for your loved one's situation.

» **Use warm packs to control pain.** Avoid electric heating pads, which may cause burns with prolonged use. Microwaveable or air-activated heat wraps offer a safer heat.

» **Use ice packs after acute injuries** sustained during falls or other accidents to reduce pain and swelling.

» **Consider massage** to aid circulation and decrease muscle soreness.

» **Add cushions as needed for comfort and support.** Avoid the use of too many pillows, which contribute to a flexed posture.

» **Be aware that increased wandering, agitation or unexplained crying in someone with dementia may be a sign of pain.**

» **See a physical therapist** for specific pain evaluation and additional recommendations.

» **Get a referral to palliative care.** Palliative care focuses on providing relief from symptoms to improve quality of life. It is appropriate at any stage of Parkinson's (from diagnosis through advanced disease). It does not mean withdrawing treatment.

Activities at Home

Advanced PD symptoms often decrease one's ability to participate in leisure activities and hobbies. Mood and thinking changes can also affect your loved one's interest in participating in the daily routine. The person with Parkinson's may feel fatigue or have a loss of motivation to try things he or she used to enjoy. It is important to encourage physical, mental and social activity whenever possible to maximize mobility and quality of life.

Keeping Active: Movement and Exercise

Regular exercise helps people with Parkinson's retain flexibility, improve circulation and maintain their abilities to complete daily tasks. It is important to practice speech, too. If you do not have time to complete regular exercise and speech practice with the person with Parkinson's, enlist the help of another family member, friend or care provider.

» **Work with a physical or occupational therapist** to design an appropriate exercise program.

» **Work with a speech pathologist** to design an appropriate breathing and speech practice program.

» **Encourage regular movements of arms and legs as part of the daily routine.** It may be necessary to split exercise into several short sessions, or to incorporate a few exercise activities during dressing or bathing tasks.

» **Focus on maintaining large, exaggerated motions whenever possible.**

» **Use small, inexpensive equipment** like balls or balloons during exercise activities to help stimulate movement.

» **Have the person with Parkinson's stand or walk with assistance** whenever possible to maintain leg strength and strong, healthy bones.

» **Engage the person with Parkinson's in daily activities that involve movement to music** (dancing, marching, singing, swaying, etc.).

» **Give no more assistance than is needed with daily activities.** Let the person help with tasks, however small, that he or she can still do.

» **Practice frequently used words or phrases**, focusing on maintaining loudness.

Keeping Active: Thinking and Memory

PD's impact on visual and thinking skills may alter the person's interests and abilities. At the same time, familiar activities can help provide stimulation and a sense of comfort.

» **Stimulate thinking skills** by encouraging the person with Parkinson's to read or listen to news or current events.

» **Place meaningful objects** like photographs and mementos in clear view to inspire and share memories.

» **Listen to audiobooks**, though concentration may limit this activity to brief intervals.

» **Encourage visits from family, friends and neighbors** to offer conversation and stimulation throughout the day.

» **Watch game shows, sporting events or nature and history programs on TV** to provide mental stimulation.

» **Try games or puzzles**, but tailor these to your loved one's situation to minimize frustration.

» **Familiar tasks** like folding towels or sorting mail may be enjoyed, even when not completed "perfectly."

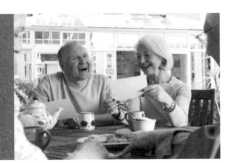

WATCH THE VIDEO

Activities at Home

Online at Parkinson.org/videos in the "CareMAP How-to Videos" playlist

Travel and Transportation

Leaving the home for medical appointments, family events or other activities can be a cumbersome process for a person with advanced-stage Parkinson's. These outings are sometimes needed, and often add to quality of life, so it is important to consider methods that promote safety and decrease caregiver stress.

Traveling to Medical Appointments

» **Try to schedule appointments at times when the person with Parkinson's is rested** and PD medications are most likely to be working well.

» If endurance allows, **schedule a few appointments on the same day**, especially if they are located in the same clinic or medical complex.

» **Pack a small bag** with your loved one's pill box, liquids, snacks and/or incontinence pads if you will be away from home for a while.

» **Make sure that the person with Parkinson's is adequately dressed for the climate** when leaving the house. Regardless of weather, you might want to bring a small shawl or lap blanket.

Getting In and Out of the House

» **Outside stairways should have sturdy railings in place.**

» **If the person with Parkinson's cannot negotiate steps, consider installing a ramp.** Make sure you work with a professional who understands the slope needed for safe walking or wheelchair transport – it should not be too steep.

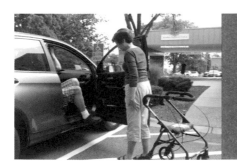

WATCH THE VIDEOS

Travel and Transportation, Parts 1 and 2

Online at Parkinson.org/videos in the "CareMAP How-to Videos" playlist

Travel by Car

Your car will likely be your main form of transportation, so it is important to be comfortable and capable of getting the person with Parkinson's and his or her assistive devices into and out of the vehicle.

» **Make sure the person with Parkinson's moves close to the car with proper body alignment**, turning to sit down safely on the car seat before attempting to move legs into the car. *(For a demonstration, watch the video "Travel and Transportation Part 1" in the "CareMAP: How-to Videos" playlist at Parkinson.org/videos.)*

» **Place a slippery satin-based fabric square or cushion on the car seat** to make it easier for the person with Parkinson's to move and get positioned.

» **Obtain adaptive equipment** to make car travel easier:

    – A portable handle can be slid into place to serve as an arm rest, allowing "push off" during transfers.

    – A seat belt hand grasp allows the person to more easily reach across and grab the belt to pull it across the body.

    – A seat belt extender makes the seat belt easier to align and lock into place.

» **Practice putting your loved one's walker or wheelchair into the trunk or back seat** of your vehicle before the day of the outing to make sure you know how to lift it safely. Practice will also make sure it fits in your car. Electric wheelchairs or scooters are generally not portable enough to be stored in a standard car trunk, which may limit the ability to use them outside the home. Some people choose to rent or buy a larger vehicle and install an electric lift, but these are expensive and not an option for everyone.

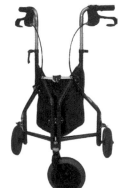

» **Consider getting a walker you can fold for transport and a transport wheelchair for outings.** Transport chairs are lighter and more portable than standard wheelchairs but are not designed to be used for heavy or continual use.

» **A physical therapist** can help you find the right items and show you how to use and lift them.

Using Medical Transportation Services

If the person with Parkinson's needs to stay in his or her wheelchair for transport, consider contacting a medical transportation service to get to appointments. These services are available in many parts of the country, and some offer sliding fee scales based on your financial situation. Most services will allow one family member to accompany the person during transport.

» **Take time to learn the company's processes** for scheduling, pick-up and drop-off service.

» **Keep the company's contact information with you** and call promptly when you are ready to go home. Be prepared for some waiting time. Make sure you have your loved one's pill boxes and other essentials in case the ride is late.

Travel by Plane

Airline travel requires pre-planning. Make sure you know all the details before setting out.

» **Call ahead** to make sure you get aisle or bulkhead seats if you need the extra space.

» **Make arrangements ahead of time** for transport assistance to your gate.

» **Avoid checking walkers or wheelchairs with luggage.** Use them until you arrive at the gate, and request that they be returned to you when you exit the plane.

» **Be prepared for travel delays:** always carry extra medications and other essentials in your carry-on luggage.

» **Tell the gate agent you need extra time to get seated.** You will usually be allowed to board first.

Special Events

While it may be difficult to get there, family events and other social activities can maximize quality of life and keep connections strong for the person with PD.

» **Before you go**, make sure the destination is accessible and support is available during the visit.

» **Enlist other family members and friends** to help arrange transportation.

» **Consider a shorter visit** to avoid fatigue, or make sure there is an opportunity to rest when needed.

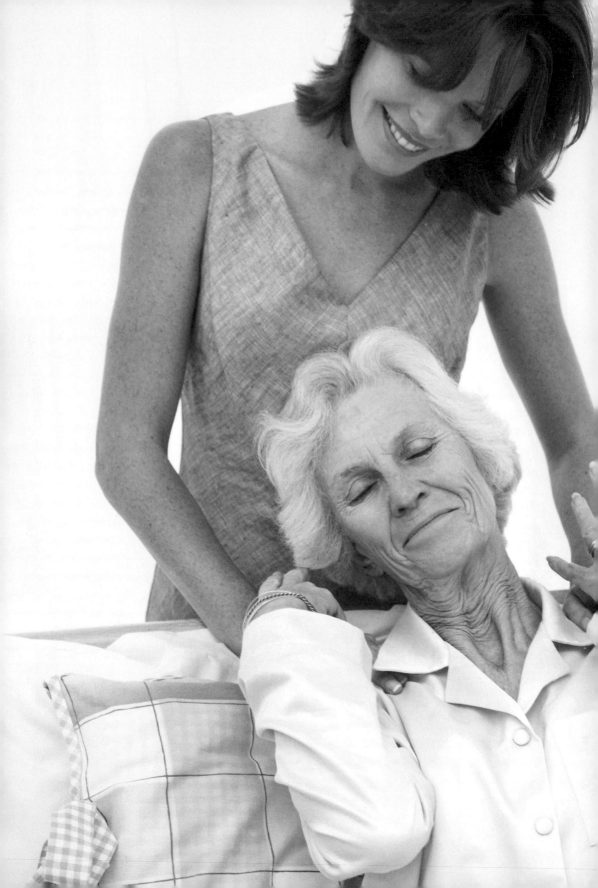

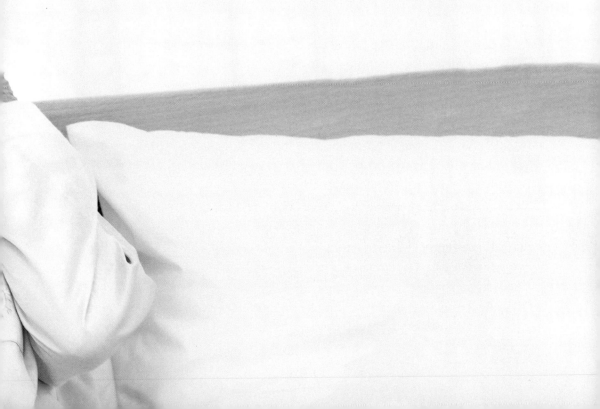

Never underestimate the power of a loving touch.

Show affection and find intimacy in caring tasks such as bathing or massage to relieve constipation.

Rest and Sleep

Getting adequate rest and sleep is an important component of overall health and quality of life. Parkinson's disease creates many challenges to getting a good night's rest, both for the person with Parkinson's and the caregiver. If your loved one is not sleeping, it is highly likely that your sleep pattern will be disrupted as well.

Bed Set-up

There are many considerations when designing ideal sleeping arrangements for you and the person with Parkinson's.

» **Choose a bed that is comfortable and conducive to sleep.**

» **Consider twin beds or sleeping in separate rooms** to ensure better rest for both you and the person with Parkinson's.

» **Use a call button, alert system or monitor** to hear the person with Parkinson's when sleeping in another room.

» **Use a firm mattress** to make rolling and movements easy to perform. Avoid water beds or excessively soft mattresses that hinder your loved one's ability to roll or move.

» **The bed height needs to allow the person to get his or her feet on the floor easily.** Removing bed casters can lower the bed to a more manageable height.

» **Obtain a half side rail or bed pole** for the person with Parkinson's to use as a sturdy hand grip when rolling or when trying to get into and out of bed.

» Rolling and moving in bed can often be made easier by using **a piece of slippery, satin-based fabric** through the middle third of the bed, so it fits under the person's shoulders and hips.

» **Avoid flannel sheets and nightwear that add friction**; these make bed movement more difficult.

» **Remove the top sheet; instead, use a lightweight comforter** to allow the person with Parkinson's to move more easily and prevent feet from becoming tangled.

» **Hospital beds can also be used to make adjustments more easily.** They can be raised during dressing and bathing and lowered as the person tries to get up.

Getting Into Bed

For demonstrations of how to help the person with Parkinson's get into and out of bed, watch the video "Rest and Sleep Part 2" in the "CareMAP: How-to Videos" playlist at www.Parkinson.org/videos.

» **Provide cues** to help the person with Parkinson's properly align her body when getting into bed.

» **Make sure the backs of both your loved one's legs are against the bed before sitting down.**

» **Help the person with Parkinson's bring her legs up as she lies down**, making an effort to stay in good alignment.

» **Avoid having the person attempt to crawl into bed** by placing a knee up on the mattress. This makes it difficult to achieve necessary alignment.

Getting Out of Bed

» When helping the person with Parkinson's out of bed, it is usually best to **start on her back**, looking up toward the ceiling.

» **Bend her knees,** allowing feet to rest firmly on the mattress. If the person with Parkinson's has a lot of morning stiffness, move the knees side to side from this position to help her become more flexible and ready to get up.

» **Help her onto her side.** Have her reach across the body to grasp the side rail or bed pole for better leverage.

» Once on the side, **help her get her feet off the bed** and begin to push up on the side rail or bed pole, moving to a seated position

» **A physical therapist** can instruct you on proper techniques to perform these transfers.

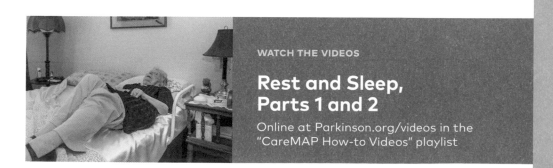

WATCH THE VIDEOS

Rest and Sleep, Parts 1 and 2

Online at Parkinson.org/videos in the "CareMAP How-to Videos" playlist

Sleep Environment

» Make sure your loved one **avoids caffeine and does not discuss stressful topics or watch loud or disturbing television programs** just before bedtime.

» **Set the bedroom temperature at a comfortable level.**

» **Try to reduce interruptions and excessive noise.**

» **Use recorded nature sounds or white noise** to achieve a more restful environment.

» **Remove objects that may cause excessive shadows** or be misinterpreted in a darkened room.

» **Talk to the doctor** if the person with Parkinson's has tremor, stiffness or mobility changes during the night that make it uncomfortable to sleep, or if she experiences frequent nightmares or hallucinations.

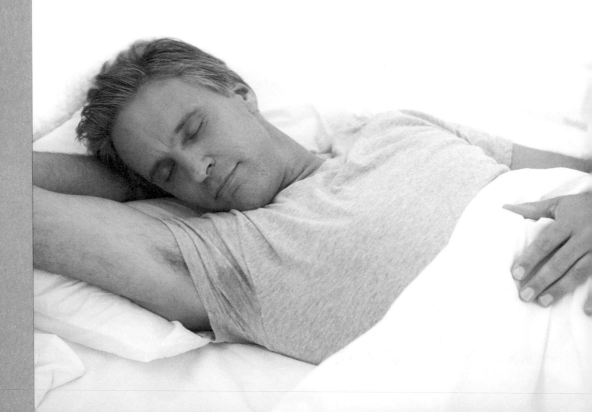

End of Life Planning

Physician Orders for Life-Sustaining Treatment (POLST)

The POLST (Physician Orders for Life-Sustaining Treatment) form is for people with serious illness or frailty where their physician would not be surprised if they died within the year. It is used in addition to the healthcare power of attorney and is meant to assure patients and their families that healthcare professionals will provide only the treatments that the patients themselves wish to receive. Most US states have a POLST program established or in development.

The POLST form acts as standing medical orders and applies to all healthcare personnel (e.g., EMTs, emergency room personnel, etc.) and in all settings (homes, assisted living facilities, nursing homes, etc.). The form is completed after a careful discussion between the doctor, patient, caregiver and any other relevant parties. The form has three sections: cardiopulmonary resuscitation (CPR), medical interventions and artificially administered nutrition.

Artificial Nutrition and Hydration (ANH) in Advanced Parkinson's Disease

Given the usual slow progression of PD, patients and families often put off what they view as the difficult discussion of whether or not artificial nutrition and hydration (ANH) should be used if swallowing problems and/or advanced dementia keep the person with Parkinson's from eating and drinking normally. Without the discussion, however, a crisis situation can develop. If the person with Parkinson's is unable to make his or her wishes known, then it is left to the healthcare power of attorney to decide whether or not to place a feeding tube.

If the person with Parkinson's is still competent and able to make care decisions, the question of whether or not to accept ANH can be made based on individual circumstances and beliefs. The patient can choose no nutrition by tube, defined trial period of tube nutrition, or long-term artificial nutrition by tube. But what if the person with Parkinson's is no longer able to make personal decisions and has not previously completed a healthcare power of attorney? The person acting as the health decision surrogate (spouse/partner, adult child, sibling, relative or close friend) may struggle with the ANH decision and not have much time to think about it. The following information may help.

If ANH is suggested because the patient is at risk for aspirating or has had a bout of aspiration pneumonia, it is important to know that the feeding tube will not prevent bacteria-laden saliva and nasal secretions from getting into the lungs and causing infection. Studies have shown that between 20-30% of elderly PD patients die of pneumonia.

Placing a feeding tube in a severely demented person can result in the patient trying to pull the tube out and needing to be physically restrained. This can worsen any agitation the person might have and may lead to the use of sedative medications. In a review of tube feeding for people with advanced dementia, the Cochrane Collaboration found no evidence that tube feeding improved quality of life. In fact, they found some evidence that tube feeding increased mortality and morbidity and reduced quality of life.

Decision-makers also worry that by not choosing ANH they are dooming the patient to a long and painful death. Reports from conscious dying patients indicate that thirst and appetite decrease naturally at the end of life. Conscious elderly patients slip quickly into a coma that is free of pain, while observation of unconscious patients indicates that the dying process is quite peaceful. If the body is shutting down in preparation for death, artificial hydration – the process of giving intravenous fluids – can actually cause distress. The body is unable to rid itself of excess fluids, which can build up in the lungs, making it hard to breath.

Ultimately, there is a difference between a person who dies because he stops eating and drinking and one who stops eating and drinking because of the natural dying process.

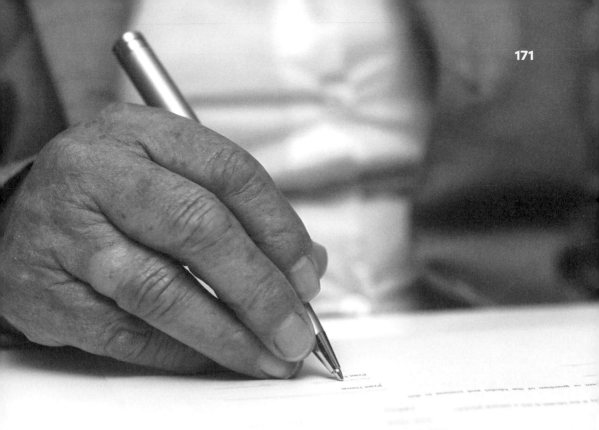

Roger and I did our end-of-life care conversations, we set up our healthcare directives with a social worker. We made our two daughters healthcare powers of attorney. We talked about each stage as it was happening, although it got harder to explain to Roger what was happening. But by talking about it we were able to adapt to each thing that came along. We also bought cemetery plots, we went over and picked them out, and it wasn't an unpleasant experience all. It's like shopping! Every once in a while we would say, 'Let's drive by our graves.' It's an odd thing to do but actually probably very healthy.

– LENNORE, CARED FOR HUSBAND, ROGER

Palliative and Hospice Care

Many people understand hospice or end-of-life care, but the term "palliative care" can still be unfamiliar. Both palliative and hospice care can provide services to assure the highest quality of life and, when the time comes, the best possible end-of-life care. The information here will help you to better understand the differences between the two and make informed choices for care. By learning about and discussing the available options before they are needed, people with Parkinson's and family members can make careful, thoughtful decisions instead of being pressured or rushed during a stressful or crisis situation.

Palliative Care

The National Hospice and Palliative Care Organization defines palliative care as patient- and family-centered care that optimizes quality of life by anticipating, preventing and treating suffering. Palliative care involves not only care of physical needs, but also the emotional, social and spiritual needs of patients, family members and caregivers. Palliative care stresses patient autonomy, access to information and choice, and it can be delivered from time of diagnosis through end of life, as a complement to other treatments.

Studies have shown that people who receive palliative care report less pain and other adverse symptoms like nausea or shortness of breath. In addition, patients report that they communicate better with their doctors and family members and experience more emotional support. Studies have also shown that palliative care ensures that care is more in line with people's wishes and meets their emotional and spiritual needs.

Palliative care is usually provided by a team of professionals that may include doctors, nurses, social workers, chaplains, pharmacists, nutritionists, counselors and others. Most insurance plans cover all or part of the palliative care treatment costs. If the patient is an enrolled veteran, palliative (and hospice) care are part of the Standard Medical Benefits Package if the need for clinical service requirement is met. If you are worried about the cost of this type of treatment, the social worker from the palliative care team can help answer your questions. The palliative care team can help patients and family members make decisions about treatment options in advanced disease and can segue into hospice care if that is desired.

Hospice

Hospice is not giving up on life or withdrawing care, nor is it a form of physician-assisted suicide. Rather, it is an approach to treatment that recognizes death as the natural ending to life and provides the person with Parkinson's the maximum amount of autonomy, dignity and comfort during the dying process.

Medicare has established three eligibility criteria for entering hospice care, and most other insurers use these as well: 1) The patient must have a life-limiting illness, and the physician must determine that to the best of his or her knowledge, the patient has six months or less to live. 2) The patient (or the healthcare power of attorney) must accept hospice rather than curative care. 3) The services must be provided by a Medicare-approved hospice program. As mentioned above, Veterans are covered under the Veterans Health Administration Standard Medical Benefits Package.

Hospice services are not actually limited to six months, though. At designated intervals, a doctor can certify that eligibility criteria continue to be met, so the person in the final phase of life can receive care for as long as necessary.

People with Parkinson's can receive hospice services wherever they reside – home, assisted living facility, skilled nursing facility or even in the hospital, but this will require two payor sources. For example, if the patient has Medicare and state-funded (Medicaid) or private insurance, one source will pay for hospice and the second one will pay for room and board at the hospital or other facility (or you will have to pay out-of-pocket). The hospice care team consists of many of the same professionals included in the palliative team, but may also include integrative therapists (massage, art, music) and volunteers.

Because PD is a chronic and progressive disease with an individualized course, it can be difficult to determine when the end of life is near. However, hospice may be appropriate if the person has symptoms such as advanced dementia, recurrent pneumonia, weight loss, urinary incontinence, infections and pain. Unfortunately, there are still some doctors who are not well versed in hospice services. If you request hospice instead of aggressive treatment, you may contact the hospice provider of your choice. The hospice will work with the treating physician to obtain the necessary referral.

When Caregiving Ends

Because Parkinson's disease is a progressive, degenerative illness, you have probably already experienced losses and the grief that follows. Loss of mobility, loss of independence, loss of his or her "former self" – grieving these losses has prepared you in some ways to grieve this final loss.

There is no set time period for grief and no right or wrong way to experience it. Initially you may feel numb and wonder if there is something wrong with you. There isn't. As time passes you will most likely experience a wide range of emotions including deep sadness, relief that the suffering for both of you has ended, loneliness and even anger. Grieving is not a staged or linear process. You may believe you have come through it, only to be struck all over again by something as simple as a familiar smell or the sight of a stranger on the street who reminds you of your loved one.

Is there life after caregiving? Yes, but things will never go back to how they were before Parkinson's. The person you cared for played a unique role in your life that no one else will ever fill, and you are not the same person that existed before you became a caregiver. Because of the all-consuming job that caregiving can be, you may need to re-establish relationships with friends and family members. You may even encounter some resentment that all your energy and attention went to the person with Parkinson's. Remember that no one who has not gone through the caregiving process will ever really be able to understand what it is like.

What can help you navigate this new chapter of your life? If caregiving chores took up most of your day, it is important to establish new routines with activities that are meaningful to you. Try to schedule several activities each week where others depend on you to show up. Volunteering, babysitting, Bible study or joining a committee working for change in your community are just some ideas – you can probably come up with many more based on your own interests and values.

These suggestions can also be helpful:

- **Be creative.** Journaling, photography, painting, wood working and crafting can be wonderful outlets for healing from loss.

- **Consider continuing to attend your PD support group.** Many people who attended a support group with their loved one find that continuing to attend the group for several months helps them transition away from their caregiver role. Others might find healing by taking on a leadership role in the group.

- **Join a bereavement support group or seek out individual grief counseling.** For some people, working with an individual grief counselor or joining a support group can help them feel less alone in the grieving process. If after a period of time you don't feel your grief lessening, you should definitely seek professional help.

- **When you are ready, remember the positive.** Once you have taken some time to heal, think about all the fun, happy moments you shared with your loved one. Consider making a memory book with pictures and stories about the person with Parkinson's that you can share with family and friends in the future.

For me, the biggest challenge of caregiving has been changing from care partnering to really becoming full-time. In the last 15 years, I've learned that I had to give up a lot of things. It wasn't really a major challenge, it's just what was needed.

The biggest reward as a caregiver? It's a little hard to choose. But probably, the biggest one is being able to return a little bit of what my wife has given to me, and to our children and our grandchildren and communities that we've lived in over so many years – to be able to return a little bit of that.

– LYLE, CARES FOR WIFE, LAVON

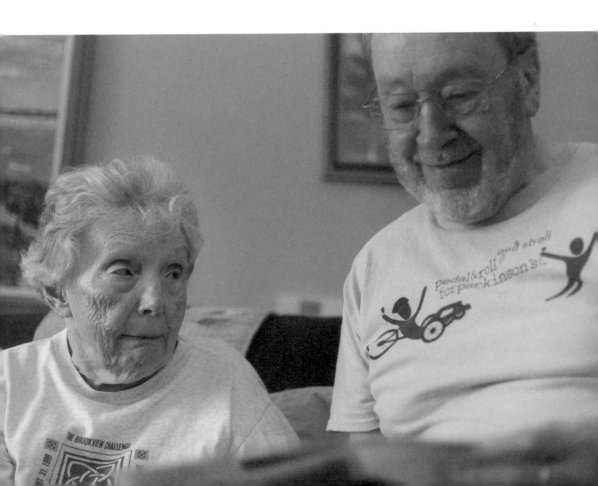